The Daily Soul Sessions
For The Pregnant Mama

A Daily Dose of Soul and Inspiration for all Thrilled, Shocked,
Excited, and Delighted Mamas To Be!

By Kacey Coppola Morreale
with Kate Coppola Leiva
& Kara Coppola Schmahl

Content and Copy Editor: Kara Schmahl
Cover Design: Ana Grigoriu www.books-design.com
Interior Illustrations: S.M. Pack, PaperBird designs on Etsy
Author Photo: Sarah Guibord

www.TheDailySoulSessions.com
TheDailySoulSessions@gmail.com

Ordering Information:
Orders by U.S. trade bookstores and wholesalers.
Please visit CreateSpace.com

Published in the United States of America
ISBN-13: 978-1519277701
ISBN-10: 1519277709

First Edition

The Daily Soul Sessions and its materials are not intended to treat,
diagnose, cure, or prevent any pregnancy or non-pregnancy related
issues. All material in The Daily Soul Sessions is provided for
inspirational purposes only. Always seek the advice of your physician
or other qualified health care provider with any questions you have
regarding a medical condition, and before undertaking any diet,
exercise, or other health program.

For Stella, JJ, and Sloane.

There would be no book without you...

Mama Love...

The Daily Soul Sessions is a special project that helps comfort and celebrate mothers-to-be with refreshing wit and spiritual depth. I wish I had stopped googling all my symptoms during my pregnancy and instead enjoyed the weird and wonderful miracle; this book helps pregnant women do just that. The lyrical and honest tone had me smiling and nodding throughout, and thinking beyond just the awkward changes to my body. I can't think of a better gift to a soon-to-be mother than to help her cherish herself at the start of this very special journey.

~Rachel Jansen, Genevieve's Mama
Account Manager, British Vogue

There is a lot of material out there for pregnant women but not much that simply acknowledges the changes, challenges and little miracles we experience daily without giving advice and listing all the "what not to do's". Reading The Daily Soul Sessions was like sitting with that friend who makes you laugh and says the right thing when you need to hear it. And I loved recognizing the different perspectives and voices from the awesome mamas that wrote the book!

~Ann Williams, Brennan and Regan's Mama
Jeweler (evermoreco.com)
& budding food entrepreneur (Momnomfoods.com)

The Daily Soul Sessions is the perfect book for any mom-to-be. During pregnancy so many women get wrapped up in all things baby; what to expect when the baby arrives and how to take care of the baby, that they often lose sight of their own needs. In just a short passage each day, The Daily Soul Sessions reminds us to take a minute for ourselves to become the best possible woman and mama that we can be.

~Kate LaMaster Mruczkowski, Carter and Grant's Mama
Creative Manager at Curb Music Publishing

Being pregnant is hard - whether you have an "easy" pregnancy or an epically challenging one. These daily inspirations are just that - inspirations. The Coppola sisters have created a pause button for you to enjoy each day in your pregnancy journey. Reminders that you are still you, that you should celebrate the beauty that is you, and that you are literally creating life and what that means are at the heart of this book. This isn't a "what to expect" book - this is a "remember to feel" book. Enjoy it. Take a moment each day to celebrate you, mama. These ladies have created a truly wonderful and enriching space for you to breathe in.

~Katie Maltais, Genevieve's Mama
Manager of Theatre

Kacey, Kate and Kara's words reach out from the pages and pet my soul. From the initial excitement of the true miracle that I was pregnant, to reminding yourself to be thankful and embrace the growth, not losing yourself - since you've lost all control and rights to your body to the baby, and curb walking. Oh, yes, curb walking is what set my little guy into motion. These women are bravest of ladies who put honesty and heart felt truth before what is "typically happening" at a milestone. FINALLY, views and experiences that make me feel like I'm sane and confirm that I am a good mama, though flawed - because aren't we all! I will definitely be adding this resource into helping my mama clients in combination with essential oils.

~Tiffany Walsh, Stuart's Mama
doTERRA Essential Oil Wellness Advocate

Introduction

I searched forever for inspiration to get me through nine months of pregnancy. Sure, there were all kinds of websites, books, and blogs, but most of what I found was very clinical. Everything either focused on the baby - *what size fruit it was each week* - or on my physical body - *how many stretch marks should I be expecting that month?!* You know, the fun stuff. But being pregnant challenged my identity on a daily basis. I suddenly didn't know where I fit into the world, what my place was. Everything changes so fast and so much, it's hard to keep up, and I needed inspiration to focus my thoughts...to help me to live in a better space every day. It may sound a little selfish, but I needed something that was a bit more about *me*, so I could become the best *me* while growing this beautiful new life inside. I couldn't find it out there, so I suddenly found myself creating it.

I've been a songwriter for the past 15 years of my life. The art of writing a song is in the three minutes it takes to tell a story, to change the life of the person listening in some small way. I write about life, its struggles, its miracles, its magic. And during those nine months, my three-minute songs became meditations, became prayers.

Every day of my pregnancy I acknowledged the obstacles I was facing, and I found ways to ride the waves. My sisters - one had just had her baby, and the other was due the same time as me - jumped right in with me, and nine months later a book was born! Every pun intended.

This book is a reminder to live each day in the moment, forget the past, and focus on the positive. It's not a "how-to", or a guide to have the perfect pregnancy. It's inspiration...a spiritual cup of coffee for the exact phase of *your* pregnancy. It's a **daily dose of soul,** so you'll greet every day grinning at the world, spewing light and life until everyone around you wants to know your secret.

These are The Daily Soul Sessions. Welcome, Mama...

First Trimester

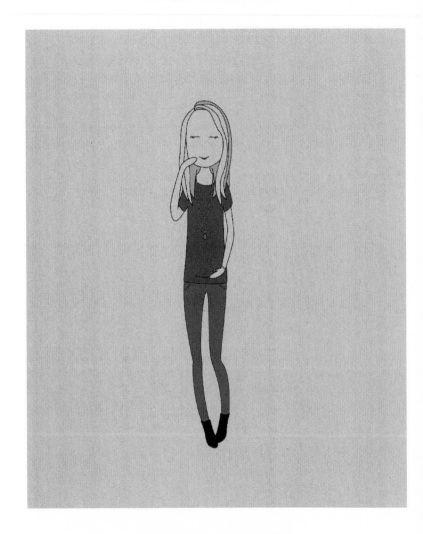

Week 1 – Week 13

The Daily Soul Sessions For The Pregnant Mama

Day 1

Pregnancy is not new to this world. But it is new *to you.*

Welcome to The Daily Soul Sessions for the Pregnant Mama-to-be. Whether you're brand new to this whole "making a baby" thing or you already have little ones, I'm so glad to be going on this journey with you! This book is meant to inspire you, to comfort you, to challenge you as you go through *tremendous* change over the next nine months. What a jaw dropping thought that is. So go ahead, take this book with you as you leap off the cliff and soar on this new adventure. After all - adventures are what life is made of - every single kicking, screaming, babbling one of them...

It's only day one. You're not even pregnant yet...but in two weeks you will be.

2 Weeks

Step one: Get pregnant. Ha. It sounds so easy doesn't it? But what can we focus on, what can we put our energy toward to help this step get accomplished? Yogis believe the body has seven chakras, or energy points throughout the body. The second chakra in our bodies is the sacral chakra, and it is located in the pelvic region. This chakra seeks pleasure and physical experience in life. Fertility originates in this part of the feminine body, as does creativity. So get creative…go create a life today.

2 Weeks, 1 Day

"The mind which is created quick to love, is responsive to everything that is pleasing, soon as by pleasure it is awakened into activity."
~Dante Alighieri, <u>The Divine Comedy</u>

Activity. Sex. Baby. One thing leads to the next right now. And it all begins with love.

"The mind... is created... to love." So get to lovin', Mama.

2 Weeks, 2 Days

"No particle can grow to seedling from anything but the whole. You know this. Why this continuous personal critique?"
~Rumi, 13th century Persian Poet, Theologian

An interesting thought as you start to make a new life.

2 Weeks, 3 Days

Chakras were first mentioned in the ancient Hindu texts of knowledge, dating back to 1500 BC. The word chakra means wheel, and many translate it to mean a "spinning wheel of light". There are seven centers or Chakras of spiritual power in the human being.

Spirit. Energy. Chi. Prana. Life. They're all the same, and they're all moving through you - and now your baby - in an endless dance from chakra to chakra. The second chakra is associated with fertility, and it is located in the pelvic region. It is also associated with the color orange. Work to loosen your hips and all the muscles surrounding as you are trying to get pregnant. Free up the space in this chakra so you have room for something new to take root.

Try practicing the yoga pose "Thread the Needle" for releasing your hips: Lie down on your back, and place your left ankle over your bent right knee. Reach through and gently pull the right knee back toward you as you breathe slowly in and out. Repeat on the other side. Imagine a big, bright orange ball of light swirling around your pelvic region as you open up and breathe.

2 Weeks, 4 Days

"Think you can, think you can't, either way you're right."
~Henry Ford

I have always loved this quote. It makes me feel brave when I lack courage. It makes me feel strong when I am confused. It makes me believe in any dream I have, and it makes me want to go after that dream with joy, determination, and beautiful optimism. If your dream is this baby…go after it.

2 Weeks, 5 Days

Whether this pregnancy is planned or not, it is happening. You are the catalyst, the cocoon for something the world has not yet seen before. The Greek Philosopher Socrates said:

"The secret of change is to focus all of your energy, not on fighting the old, but on building the new."

What are you fighting to let go of today so that you can pour all of your energy into this new chapter in the story of your life?

Getting pregnant can either take a short time or a long one. Every person on this planet has a different experience with it. Maybe that is why we don't talk about it a lot until it happens. My experience will be completely my own. And yours will be yours. The one thing we do have control over is our thoughts. How we look at each day, each month as we start this process. I choose positivity, light, and optimism. What do you choose?

"A pessimist sees the difficulty in every opportunity; an optimist sees the opportunity in every difficulty."
~Winston Churchill

3 Weeks

"Do not conform any longer to the pattern of this world, but be transformed by the renewing of your mind."
~Romans 12:2

Life is what we make of it. Creating a new life is what we make of it. Just because the world says it is one way does not mean it must be that way for you. Stay mindful, stay in the moment, renew your perspective, and be transformed...

3 Weeks, 1 Day

Before you take the test and find out if you're pregnant or not, it's hard to know for sure. I would have sworn I was experiencing normal PMS, "about to get my period" symptoms. But then you pee on the stick, hold your breath...and squeal in disbelief, excitement, nervous shock, *whatever* - and suddenly realize these symptoms were so much more than normal. Not to mention the boobs...have you *noticed* your boobs? It's mind boggling how fast they can change. So. What symptoms do you have today?

3 Weeks, 2 Days

Now is such a good time to start a journal. Do you write? Draw? Doodle? Scrapbook? This is one of the most interesting times of your life, and in the grand scheme of things, a very short one too. So fill the pages with your thoughts, dreams, ideas, fears, and faith. One day you may love looking back through it...or perhaps it's just a perfect way to settle your mind and start your day.

3 Weeks, 3 Days

Chakra Crash Course...here's the deal. Yogis believe our bodies are filled with energy. There are seven points throughout the body, where the energy pools and moves on. Starting at the "root" and moving up to the "crown" of the head, the energy begins with the most basic of everyday securities: safety, physical identity, ambition, and all the way up to inspiration, spirituality, and connection with the divine.

It's interesting to take stock of your life, where you are at, where you feel stuck, where you feel free. Meditating, saying a prayer, being aware of the stagnant aspects of your life can truly help to open you up and live in the moment of today... and everyday.

3 Weeks, 4 Days

"And suddenly you know. It's time to start something new, and trust the magic of beginnings."
~Meister Eckhart, German Theologian, Philosopher, Mystic

Beginners luck - you've heard it before. If you're a beginner at this growing a baby thing...take heart. We've got luck on our side. That and we simply don't know what's in store for the next nine months. But that is exciting...who wants to know the end of the story before they get there anyway?

3 Weeks, 5 Days

Before a long journey, I always visualize the place I am going. I love to paint a picture in my mind of the adventures yet to come. A little positive affirmation and visualization never hurt anyone. So I see myself wherever I am going: on the vacation, in the new house, holidays with family. Creating memories, living life. This new journey is rather difficult to visualize though. It is hard to see what I have never seen before. But I'll try. Endless blessings on this new journey, Mama. Let's go on it together...

3 Weeks, 6 Days

"Face with all our courage what is now to be"
~W.H. Auden "Geography of the House." A Poem

Chilling. Beautiful. Lovely. It reminds me to put my big girl pants on this morning and get excited about the endless blessings of this day.

What is a Mother?

Discovering that you are going to have a baby is shocking whether you are planning it or not. When I saw that little positive sign in the pee stick, I was shell shocked to say the least. But after that initial deer in the headlights feeling, I can't get a certain word out of my head...*Mother*. I am going to be a *mother*. And so are you...just let that word swirl around for a little while. It means so many things in so many ways.

4 Weeks, 1 Day

Meditation: Calming Anxiety and Fear

You are on a train, and it is taking you somewhere new, whether you're ready or not. But you cannot let fear of the unknown win over the next nine months.

Close your eyes. Start to slow your breath and feel it fill your whole body - in, out, in, out. Picture yourself standing on a vast cliff, and all you can see, all around you, is beauty, space, life. Feel the strength, not the scared. Repeat to yourself: *I am enough. I am enough. I am enough...*

Because you are. It is you, mama, who is doing the work now. And you'll get to where you're going, one way or another. Trust the process. And trust yourself.

4 Weeks, 2 Days

Do you feel like you are walking around with the BIGGEST SECRET IN THE HISTORY OF THE WORLD right now? I feel as though I may spontaneously combust any second, this secret is so big. So much feeling caused by such a small cell. Like the Big Bang Theory, I'm pretty sure I could create a new universe today. Something from nothing...more like *everything* now...

4 Weeks, 3 Days

Hangover:
a. *Disagreeable physical effects following heavy consumption of alcohol*
b. *A letdown following great excitement or excess (Merriam-Webster.com)*

HA. If only the feeling we woke up to everyday was something we could undo by not consuming that last glass of wine. The only "excess" you're experiencing now is the mass production of new cells, brains and placentas being made. But this dense fog can only be described as a constant and weary hangover these days. And unfortunately there's no hair of the dog to cure it. All praise Motherhood...and you.

4 Weeks, 4 Days

18 days after conception, your baby's heart starts beating. Imagine that. *18 days*...the cells have multiplied, and your tiny little baby has a *heart* that starts to beat.

And the miracles are just beginning...

4 Weeks, 5 Days

I didn't mean to get pregnant. There it is. Sshhhh. Don't tell anyone lest the judgment begin. The eye roll, the knowing smirk, the "You didn't mean to, but you didn't *mean* to?", "Do you even *know* how babies get made?", "You know the pull and pray method doesn't really work, right?". Sigh. Yes. To all those statements. I know it happens, and it is still mind-numbingly *shocking* when you've spent your whole life *not being pregnant,* to suddenly and heart-stoppingly *find yourself pregnant.* Alas. That is my story. It begins with a dirty martini and a pee stick - or a beer garden and a pizza - both were memorable...

What was your heart stopping *I'm pregnant* moment? Write it down. Remember it. Someday you'll start it with "once upon a time..." as you put your babes to bed.

Emotion. Overload. Joy, fear, excitement, shock, concern, expectation. Can you literally feel your entire life change in an instant? I do. Like a lightening bolt or a crash of thunder…this baby is changing the world. No looking back now.

5 Weeks

If everyone lived the life they dreamt of, the magic would leave a little. It wouldn't be so awe inspiring when one of us actually breaks the chains of "reality" and does something incredible. If fear no longer existed...life would become a little dull don't you think? That's part of the fun, part of the freedom, part of the seduction of dreams. The conquering of them. The knee shaking fear that you quietly tell "no" to day after day after day. And when you make one dream come true...the magic doesn't leave after all. Another dream is waiting in the wings. That is what it is to be brave.

Be brave new mama...you just made one dream come true. So what's next?

5 Weeks, 1 Day

"Am I crazy?" she asked. "I feel like I am sometimes."
"Maybe," he said, rubbing her forehead. "But don't worry about it. You need to be a little bit crazy. Crazy is the price you pay for having an imagination. It's your superpower. Tapping into the dream. It's a good thing not a bad thing."
~Ruth Ozeki, <u>A Tale for the Time Being</u>

Our Superpower. What a delicious thought for today. Let's all be superheroes, get a little crazy, and dream today. It's a wonderful gift to dream.

5 Weeks, 2 Days

The definition of *fatigue* does not begin to describe the bone deep, foggy weariness that hangs around you these days. Nothing looks different to the outside world, but inside you are so so so so so so so *tired*. Did you know that in the early days of pregnancy you are exerting the same amount of energy as you would if you were in the gym body building all day? Every day. I had to pass this information along to my husband when he looked at me incredulously at my 7 pm bedtime. This too shall pass, Mama...this too shall pass.

5 Weeks, 3 Days

So I have started to eat prunes. Yup. It was inevitable I guess, and I urge you, Mama, to start eating them daily. One of the most annoying side effects of pregnancy is constipation, especially if you have to up your iron intake. Start your regimen early...you won't regret it! My trick when they are hard to choke down? I throw them in a smoothie - the sweetness makes it extra delicious.

5 Weeks, 4 Days

Right now, today, before you lose any more control of your body, start taking care of it. Continue to exercise, stretch, and maintain your flexibility for as long as you and your Doctor say you can. Physical activity fights fatigue, is healthy for your baby, and is vital to keeping you balanced. I know it's hard to add that into an already exhausting day, but I promise we won't regret it nine months from now. Take time for you. No one else will.

5 Weeks, 5 Days

Believing in the unseen...is that what faith is? Every so often, I have these moments where I'm dubious of this whole pregnancy thing. Am I really pregnant? Really!? How many pregnancy tests have you taken, new mama? If you're like me, you took two. If you're like my best friend, you took ten. Either way, your period has gone on an open-ended vacation, and it seems you are really and truly pregnant. Don't worry; your first doctor appointment will bring proof that there is indeed a tiny miracle growing inside of you. But in the meantime, rely on your instinct, on your gut feeling that you are on your way to mamahood. And if all else fails, look at that pregnancy test again - you know you kept it!

5 Weeks, 6 Days

Meditation: Faith
Faith: *Strong belief or trust in someone or something (Merriam-Webster.com)*

Faith will get you through the early days of your pregnancy. The phrase *blind faith* didn't originate out of thin air - faith is the belief in something that we have not yet seen. It's a powerful thing, to be faithful. Today as you close your eyes and begin to breathe deeply, ask yourself where your faith lives. In your heart? In the pit of your stomach? Maybe it's in your fingertips. Wherever your faith lies, visualize a bright flame in that spot, illuminating the faith you have in yourself, in your new baby, and in the world you are creating for your family. As you breathe in, let the flame get brighter. As you breathe out, visualize that flame warming the world around you. Continue to breathe and visualize this light until your heart feels settled. Have faith, Mama.

6 Weeks

The only thing in all of creation that worries is a human being. Plants don't worry. Animals don't worry. They live in the moment, in survival mode, from second to second.

As you go through your day, try to remember this, and leave some of your panic behind. This time in your life is surreal and unreal - it's hard to actually accept that you are pregnant! But worrying all day long isn't worth it, gorgeous mama. Give that worry to God, or someone much more in control than you, and just be grateful that you are what you are. Right now. Today.

6 Weeks, 1 Day

After about a week of walking around in a fog, the idea of being pregnant becomes a little more real. I looked up the definition of mother just to see what the dictionary said it meant. Here is what I found:

Mother:

a. *A female person who is pregnant with or gives birth to a child.*
b. *A female person whose egg unites with a sperm, resulting in the conception of a child.*
c. *A woman who adopts a child.*
d. *A woman who raises a child. (Thefreedictionary.com)*

Wow...so clinical, so cut and dried, so...superficial. I guess we'll have to figure this out on our own - through our own journey. Then, maybe we can come up with our own definition.

What does *Mother* mean to you?

Meditation: Mother

What does "Mother" mean to you? What words rise to mind? Close your eyes and breathe deeply. In through your nose, out through your nose. As you breathe in think *"mo"* and as you breathe out think *"ther."*

Mo...ther...Mo....ther...Mo...ther.

Continue to breathe slowly, steadily, and mindfully. Take notice of any images or feelings that arise. Let them float around inside your mind like fallen leaves floating on a river. Don't give too much weight to any of those thoughts or feelings. Instead let them spin their way down the river...simply let them be. Try to practice this meditation a few times a week. Perhaps when you first wake up. Lie still in your bed and begin to breathe mindfully...

...Mo....ther......Mo...ther......Mo...ther....

6 Weeks, 3 Days

It's pretty mind-blowingly crazy how fast you become protective of the little peanut inside of you. It feels so new, so fleeting, so fragile. Logically we know it's early and tenuous, but how can you not worry? How can you enjoy the moment that you are in, without giving into the *what ifs?* Most say staying in the moment is the essential key to happiness. To conquering fear and doubt. Staying in the moment and choosing to smile, choosing to be brave, choosing to be happy.

6 Weeks, 4 Days

Have you told your family this crazy, exciting news yet? It's magical how loving and happy and thrilled your loved ones are when they find out. Even though the whole world doesn't know yet, the people that really matter do, and it's achingly sweet how much hope a new life brings.

6 Weeks, 5 Days

"A baby will make love stronger, days shorter, nights longer, bankroll smaller, home happier, clothes shabbier, the past forgotten, and the future worth living for."
~Pablo Picasso

6 Weeks, 6 Days

Lately I have found that it is perfectly normal to feel like superwoman one moment - *look what my body is doing!* - and like the most fragile piece of glass the next - *don't hug me, don't hug me - ahhhhh.* Take courage in this universal truth: Women have been having babies for a very, very long time. You are the next in line to join this sisterhood. You are superwoman. You are strong. You are creative. You are creating...

7 Weeks

Distraction: *extreme agitation of the mind or emotions. (Encyclopedia.com)*

Like a pinball in a machine, your thoughts and emotions are probably bouncing around from happy to sad, excited to disbelief, crying to reeling. It's so hard to concentrate on any one thing, right? Every second a million cells are dividing and growing and spinning and functioning all at once inside of you. Sometimes you feel just like one of those cells, and every second is a new one. Some people take drugs to feel this good...lucky you!

Meditation: Grounding Yourself

Lie down flat on the floor. Bonus points if you do this outside! Close your eyes, and say hello to your breath. Begin to become aware of the ground beneath you. Feel how supportive the earth is under your heels, your calves, your thighs and hips. Feel the stable ground cradling your back, shoulders, neck and head. Turn your palms flat on the floor and gently send gratitude to the earth. There is a reason why we call her Mother…she is steady and grounding…she absorbs all of your spinning emotions and gives you the support you need to continue on your journey.

7 Weeks, 2 Days

In significant times of change I have trouble focusing on individual things. My thoughts and emotions spin maddeningly around in a bubble of nervous energy. Nothing gets done. Everything seems too much, and the day is wasted on inactivity. Do you ever feel this way? That there is simply too much to do, and the finish line seems a marathon away. This is a significant time of change, so take this day one step at a time. One breath at a time. The future will make itself known then. This moment is yours for the living.

Nausea, nausea, nausea. Ugh. Did I mention the nausea? It's there. *All the time.* And what's worse...the only thing that helps it is *to eat*. It's some sort of twisted joke. Honey Nut Cheerios helped, oddly enough, when nothing else sounded remotely edible. What works for you?

7 Weeks, 4 Days

"If nothing ever changed, there'd be no butterflies."
~Author Unknown

Ahhh. Tis a scary, unknown world we are entering. But what's coming on the other side will be delicious, beautiful, and oh so worth it.

7 Weeks, 5 Days

If nothing ever changes, then *nothing ever changes*. We can either look at change as scary or wonderful. In a way, when I finally succumb to graceful change, even if it's just for today, I always find freedom. It is such a relief to ride the waves of change and see where the water takes you.

7 Weeks, 6 Days

"Acceptance is peace. It washes away the tension of what we think should be and wraps us in the ease of what is."
~Quietlotus.com

Belief, disbelief...boy, girl...known, unknown - it is far easier, far more peaceful to accept what is happening inside of you than to build expectation or try to control what is far beyond ours to control.

Acceptance is peace.

8 Weeks

Are you headed to the doctor - finally! - this week? Channel the butterflies into positive energy and get excited! Perhaps the surreal will feel more real after that first visit...and first sonogram picture!

8 Weeks, 1 Day

In Yoga, it is believed that mother and child share energy during pregnancy. Whatever mom feels, her child inherits. In these early days, it is important to make conscious daily choices as to what you want to feel, and what thoughts you let take root in your mind. Nerves, anxiety, doubt all bring chaos to that forming baby...and you!

We are cyclical beings in the world. Our lives are not linear. Everything happens in cycles and seasons - passion, creativity, wisdom, success - they all ebb and flow. Right now your fertility is taking priority. Let it. Breathe in the morning sunshine, and accept the cycle your life is in today.

8 Weeks, 3 Days

Meditation: Calming Meditation
Our bodies are made up of 60% water.

Three quarters of the Earth is covered in water.

My mother's cure for everything is to *"drink more water!"*

Water is everywhere. Water calls to our souls. We recognize it as like recognizes like. So as you close your eyes in meditation today, picture the ocean. Visualize gentle waves, continuously rolling in to kiss the beach. Hear the song they sing as they endlessly crash on the sand. It's calming, isn't it? To think of the water, to hear the waves, to know that their reliability can be a constant in your life. When you are feeling anxious or nervous or simply too excited, come back to these waves. Come back to the water. (Waterinfo.org)

Speaking of water, why don't you go ahead and drink some today? It is so good for you and your baby. Doctor it up with fresh mint, chopped strawberries, and a squeeze of lemon or lime juice for a really delicious treat! Drink up, buttercup.

8 Weeks, 5 Days

"Each morning we are born again. What we do today is what matters most."
-Buddha

In a way we are all born, over and over, everyday. It's a hopeful thought. Yesterday may have been hard, it may have been magical...either way, today is a new day. The only day that matters.

The only day we have.

Isn't it funny how you feel the highest of highs and the lowest of lows these days? The lightning quick changes in my belly and soul leave me breathless at times. But would I prefer the calm even keel of a blue sky every day? The ups and downs are what make us feel alive. Maybe the point is to not let the lows keep us down too long, and to absolutely cherish the highs when they come. Because everything is passing. Every second of every day is transforming into the next...and the next...and the next. And there is hope in that today.

9 Weeks

Disbelief: inability to accept that something is true or real.
Synonyms: incredulity, astonishment, amazement, surprise. (Google Search Definitions)

My body is strangely numb some days. What is *happening* inside this tummy of mine? Most likely you've been to the doctor - thank goodness - and confirmed that you aren't totally nutso, but it is still hard to wrap your head around the fact that there is another life growing at an incredible rate inside of you. If it weren't for the narcolepsy and the stomach grinding nausea, disbelief may win out on your emotions today. It can be astonishing how much your life is changing, and with that astonishment comes fear, excitement, weariness, or disbelief.

I sometimes feel like if I can't actually see the baby, have an ultrasound once a week, then the knowledge that I am still pregnant seems harder to hold on to. So silly...who has a weekly ultrasound?

So my quest has become this: How can I start to connect with this child - before I feel it flutter, before my tummy starts growing - how can I start to *believe* that this is happening. I'll let you know how it goes, but for now? I will simply tell myself *I am still pregnant.* I will believe. And it's only four short weeks until I see that sucker again...

9 Weeks, 1 Day

Ok. So you're pregnant - *still crazy to think, right?* - and chances are you do not know the sex of this baby yet. Cultures all around the world have come up with various traditions claiming a way to figure out the sex!

A Chinese superstition claims that a woman can influence the sex of her baby by eating certain food, usually seven days prior to conception. According to this myth, carrots, lettuce, mushrooms, and tofu can ensure the conception of a baby boy. But if a woman wants to have a girl, she should have fish, meat, and pickles. (Buzzle.com)

9 Weeks, 2 Days

Have you noticed your hormones "hormone-ing" yet? Pay attention to the cycles of the moon during these months. The Earth experiences 20% higher tides during a full moon. That is an incredible change to a vast body of water. We, as humans, are mostly water, so it's not surprising that our bodies are highly affected by the changing of the moon. Add some pregnancy hormones to that, and you've got a party.

9 Weeks, 3 Days

As much as we want to be able to see the future, no one has invented that crystal ball yet. This does not stop us from worrying and anxiously attempting to control the events in our lives on a daily basis. Right now your body has taken over, and if there is any proof of nature, God, and miracles, pregnancy is it. You cannot see what is happening inside, but have faith...you are on a magical ride.

"We live by faith, not by sight."
~2 Corinthians 5:7

9 Weeks, 4 Days

Meditation: Phases of the Moon

The moon is in a constant state of change. Phase to phase, new to full, waxing to waning. Some days the moon shows us her full, bright face in all its glory. Others, she only grants a sliver of her light. And one day a month she goes completely dark. But you know as well as I do that this doesn't mean the moon isn't there. We just can't see it from our spot on Earth. As you go about your day today, stop every now and then to think about the moon. Think about how even when we can't see her full and bright, she is still there. Apply this to your life...you haven't held your baby yet, but he is still there. A tiny light inside of you in a constant state of change. Believe in your little one as you believe in the moon. Embrace the light inside of you.

Take a nap. Just do it. Succumb to the exhaustion that envelops you these days. Pamper yourself by allowing your body to rest. There is so much work going on inside, it is okay to feel tired. And sleep is so good for you. Especially when nights are restless. Shut the office door, sneak away to your car, turn the cell phone off, and close your eyes. You'll feel like a new woman.

9 Weeks, 6 Days

You are slowly learning to share the space inside you. Before your tummy really starts to grow, it is sometimes hard to imagine a baby floating around inside. There are also so many emotions flowing through you. Are they all yours? Do some belong to the tiny life beginning to take shape? Who knows? I can only guess that this sharing of space and self never really ends once you are a mother - but that doesn't mean you have to lose yourself.

"Today you are You, that is truer than true. There is no one alive that is Youer than You."
~Dr. Seuss

Do something just for you today.

The third chakra is located in your core. It is associated with the color yellow, and it encourages individualism and a "break away from the pack" mentality. Focusing on your third chakra can help you create an identity for your pregnancy. *Your pregnancy.* How do you see it going? What do you want to feel, be, and show the world during this incredible time of change? Especially as your core literally changes - is that a bump or breakfast? Visualize a bright ball of golden light, an illuminating sun filling your third chakra and let it inspire you and the people you love.

10 Weeks, 1 Day

The third chakra is the center of your self-esteem. The coming weeks will bring challenges, but every time you judge or compare yourself to others you are depleting this chakra and causing an imbalance within. You have the power to choose and accept the challenges and changes coming your way. You have the power to choose *grace*. And acceptance. And love.

10 Weeks, 2 Days

How many fingers can you cross to maximize good luck? The next few weeks will probably come with a lot of doctor appointments, which can be stressful. Author Anne Lamott says:

"(life is) filled with heartbreaking sweetness and beauty, floods and babies and acne and Mozart, all swirled together."

Yin and yang, ebb and flow, summer and winter...they are all a part of life. Such beauty, such ugly, such life. The more we learn to gracefully endure it and stay even throughout the roller coaster ride, the happier life is.

10 Weeks, 3 Days

Meditation: Breathe in the Light

There is enough stress in your life right now, so bringing any sort of self-judgment into it is silly and extremely unproductive, don't you think? Your meditation for today is this: close your eyes and let any thoughts of self-doubt or worry that you aren't doing enough for your baby float out the nearest window. I'm serious. Send. Them. On. Their. Way. Breathe in clean, fresh air full of positive light, and breathe out any dark thoughts or feelings. Breathe in the light, breathe out the dark...breathe in light, breathe out dark...in light, out dark...in light...light.....light....

10 Weeks, 4 Days

As that baby keeps cooking and growing and taking up space inside me, I suddenly feel a little selfish. Or maybe *self-centered* is a better way of putting it. I have less energy to focus on the outside world when so much energy is focused on the inside. The smallest requests, social engagements, even dirty dishes seem like climbing a mountain. I just want to curl up and read a good book, take in a movie, cuddle with my love. And that is okay. It's okay to send all the love and energy I have to the tiny life inside...and leave the outside to themselves for today.

10 Weeks, 5 Days

In *The Book of Secrets: Unlocking the Hidden Dimensions of Your Life*, Deepak Chopra said that most people think life passes too quickly. There's not much you can do about it. But if you can find true mindfulness, and work toward practicing it every day, then life becomes single moments that refresh and become new every second that follows. Just because you were sad yesterday, does not mean you are sad today. Choose a different path...and choose better.

10 Weeks, 6 Days

"Alone had always felt like an actual place to me, as if it weren't a state of being, but rather a room where I could retreat to be who I really was."
Cheryl Strayed, <u>Wild</u>

Pregnancy. It can make you feel so alone. Even if you have an incredible support system it is still a personal journey. No one really knows exactly what your body is feeling. No one really knows the thoughts that run through your mind every waking second. No one could possibly understand those crazy dreams you've started to experience (what is *up* with those dreams anyway?).

Strayed makes being alone a not so scary place to be. Her words make "alone" feel like a sacred spot, a quiet spot, a peaceful refuge where you don't have to try so hard. Where you are free to think and say and feel exactly what you want.

So. Try to embrace the "alone-ness" you sometimes feel. Try to see it as that "room where you can retreat to be who you really are." Embrace this roller coaster, mama! And revel in your miracle working amazingness!

11 Weeks

Meditation: Ball of Light

Sit comfortably and close your eyes. Breathe in and out slowly and deeply. After a few deep breaths, settle the breath so that your inhale is the same length as your exhale. Count to 4 as you inhale and 4 as you exhale. Picture a spinning ball of light in the center of your heart. Feel light and energy pulsating out with each heartbeat. Now picture an identical ball of light in the center of your baby's heart. As you did with your own, feel that light expanding out with every beat of your little one's heart. See the spot where the light from your heart and the light from her heart meet. Convergence. Visualize these dancing balls of light shining more and more life in an ever-expanding radius. Lucky you! How blessed you are to carry your little one's light with you for these few short months - alright, long months. But short in the long run. You get it.

Shine bright, precious mama.

11 Weeks, 1 Day

Wrap your head around this: that sweet little baby inside of you is almost *fully formed*. Even if they are only four centimeters big...they are a little human doing summersaults and wriggling around. I sometimes take comfort in that thought when my energy is - surprise, surprise - lagging. Hey if we can create a fully formed human...what can't we do?! Take strength in that thought, Mama, and go conquer the world today.

11 Weeks, 2 Days

The haze of the first trimester is starting to wear off ever so slowly. Some days may actually give you hope that soon you won't want to sleep the entire day away. Do you already find yourself missing some things from your old life? That relaxing glass of wine, the third cup of coffee, Friday night sushi dates? It's kind of cliché and annoying how true the saying is - "you don't miss it 'til it's gone" - and then you cannot stop thinking about it. This first trimester is so important and fragile, it seems we treat it and ourselves the most carefully. If the nausea and exhaustion give you the night off, it's nice to slip into your old self sometimes: order a California roll, go on a date night...be yourself...it feels good.

11 Weeks, 3 Days

Although you're still deep in the secret days of the first trimester, there is a glimmer of light at the end of the tunnel. Does everyone around you think you are completely crazy by now? I feel as if I have a neon *I'm pregnant* sign tattooed on my forehead, but everyone else has yet to guess. If the amount of naps, trips to the bathroom, and moody moments don't tip them off, what possibly could? But that's the thing about pregnancy. It is the most intense, introverted nine months of your life - so accept it, and enjoy it. People will know soon enough.

11 Weeks, 4 Days

Isn't it funny how during these first three months of pregnancy, we keep this enormous secret from all the people around us? Yet it's quite possibly the time when we need the most support. Mentally and physically, you are going through the biggest changes you've *ever* experienced, but most likely only a few people in your life know. Hold on to those people. Keep them close and be sure to share your feelings with them. They are your tribe, and they want to support you. And give yourself a break, too. Go ahead and take a long nap today. You deserve it!

What does it mean to keep your heart open? In Yoga you focus so much on the heart center, on opening and expanding that area to increase the flow of energy. Ancient Chinese medicine calls that energy your *Chi*. Yogis call it *Shakti*. Christians call it the *Spirit*. All three encourage us to keep that energy open and flowing. That energy is the seed of life, of love, of every happy thought that you have in a day. Try to keep your heart open today...in every situation. When the heart closes down, that energy gets stuck, and depression and anxiety get stuck as well. Stay free. Stay happy. Stay open.

11 Weeks, 6 Days

Whatever challenges you are facing today, face them with courage. Even the smallest obstacles give way to a stronger tomorrow.

"Mindfulness meditation doesn't change life. Life remains as fragile and unpredictable as ever. Meditation changes the heart's capacity to accept life as it is."
~Sylvia Boorstein, Meditation Teacher, Psychotherapist, Storyteller

A Pregnancy superstition: If you are craving sweets, you are carrying a girl, if it's sour that you want…? It's a baby boy.

So are you into ice cream or pickles today?

12 Weeks, 1 Day

I am a warrior. You are a warrior. There is no other path around this adventure. And adventure it must be. I've found refuge in yoga during this time of enormous change in my life. Yoga grounds me, brings me back to myself, makes me see things in a calmer and bigger way. Today I learned that in times of challenge, it is our natural instinct to tense up, to contract, to freeze. To become immobile and stiff. To stop moving. And in order to survive childbirth, in order to get through this phase in my life, it is necessary, it is *vital* to fight against these natural instincts. To do the exact opposite, run as fast as I can in the other direction. To keep moving. No matter how big or how small these movements are, I must keep moving. Keep breathing and finding space inside myself, inside my life, for growth, for change, for movement. In my small little universe of pregnancy I can look at this concept and apply it to every second of my life. Not just bringing a surprising and beautiful child into the world, but also me...my life...my journey. I am a warrior. I may feel like freezing up today, contracting into a small ball. But I cannot. I must keep moving - even if it's just to my yoga mat. And through this space I create...I find acceptance, I find surprises, I find change....

...I find hope.

Meditation: Finding Space

Breath on its own creates space inside of you. Think about it - as you inhale your lungs get bigger, your chest puffs out, your stomach expands. Voila! More space. Close your eyes and deepen your breath. Feel how every breath gives you that extra, sacred space inside of you. Breathing is an art, and when we do it mindfully, we give ourselves the gift of noticing a moment of freedom, a moment of calm, a moment of space. Stringing all those breaths and moments together is the goal...and may lead to a pretty awesome nap! Happy Breathing!

12 Weeks, 3 Days

Some mornings you just need a little outside stimulation to get your day started. So here goes: today my sister happened to send me a link to a food blogger named Mimi Thorisson. I'd never heard of her so I looked up her website...and was hit with a thousand pounds of inspiration! After a career in fashion, media, and television, she and her photographer husband moved to a farmhouse/chateau in Medoc, France to raise their six kids and even more dogs and - well - basically just be fabulous. She has a passion for life, a passion for food, a passion for family, and a passion for her man. Pretty much the person I want to be when I grow up. Check her blog out - MimiThorisson.com. You will not regret it. And you may just want to book a trip to France too.

12 Weeks, 4 Days

They say good things come in threes. Let's look at that, shall we? We have the three little pigs, the three stooges...the french hens, and the Hansen Brothers. There's the BLT and Destiny's Child, the beginning, middle, and end. The Rule of Three is a writing principle that states that things that come in threes are "inherently funnier, more satisfying, and more effective than any other number" - did you see the three there?! And let's add one more...the three trimesters of pregnancy. See? All good things come in threes...(Rule of Three, Wikipedia)

12 Weeks, 5 Days

Being pregnant is one of the most *absorbing* times in your life. It's such an introverted time, and it should be. There is simply too much happening inside you to not retreat a little. But how can we focus that absorbing energy *outward* and avoid trapping ourselves in our own conflict filled mind? How can we go after what really matters? Let's embrace gratitude and love, helping friends and family, and leaving this world just a little bit better than we found it. Let's be *absorbed by life* today, Mama.

12 Weeks, 6 Days

"She is clothed with strength and dignity; and she laughs without fear of the future."
~Proverbs 31:25

I love when I come across a quote, verse, Facebook update, or a friend that says the perfect thing at the perfect time. It's kismet, destiny. There is quite a road ahead of us in the next six months. If this is your first time being pregnant, like me...you really have no idea what to expect. Even if it's your second or third or fourth time - pregnancy can still be surprising. No two humans are alike, so it's safe to say no pregnancy is alike. That can cause some sleepless nights and anxious wonder. But I still want to be like that girl...who laughs without fear of the future...don't you?

13 Weeks

AH! We're almost there. So close to the second trimester. It is so tempting to want to jump up and run, be active, celebrate. You are feeling better, the nausea has FINALLY bowed down and walked away with its tail between its legs. Everyone tells you how much better you'll feel, how much more energy you'll have. I rush to my yoga mat and try a more challenging class…

And my body betrays me. Light headed, dizzy, sudden lack of energy for even a decent down dog. We must be growing a spleen today because I can't seem to find my rhythm. Frustration emanates from my pores as I try to push through. This is wrong, my teacher tells me. You must go with what your body and baby tell you. Every day. You must accept the tired days, the draining days, just as you soar on the days when you feel like flying. *Because the only thing that doesn't change during pregnancy is the fact that everyday will.* Every day will be different. So as the class around me twists into yet another camel pose, I quiet my mind and quiet my pride…and slip into a restoring hip opener. I breathe. I accept my limitations as my body accepts astronomical change, and I enjoy this day - this phase - for exactly what it is.

If you are having a low day, read a book, grab a massage, sit in nature. Take time for you. Because after all…

…Tomorrow is another day.

13 Weeks, 1 Day

As women, we are programmed from a very young age to compare ourselves to other women. Many of us are always focused on the outside world, on what we want instead of what we have. I struggle with it more than I care to admit. Most recently I have experienced this unavoidable comparison of myself to other pregnant women. However far along they are, I can't help but notice how much my body is different from theirs.

It's a struggle. But there is no way we can go through the next six months constantly comparing ourselves to a stranger walking down the street. As women, as human beings, we all have our daily challenges. And I realize - I have *no idea* what struggles that stranger has in *her* life. How dare I put her on a pedestal and forget to just love her like a sister despite all the insecure comparisons. I have to work on letting go of comparing myself to anyone else. And this is my challenge to you, sister. *Let Go.* Because if you really think about it…holding on is just a waste of our precious time.

13 Weeks, 2 Days

Meditation: Sisterhood

Think of a woman in your life. Perhaps one who is pregnant as well, or trying to be, or just had her baby. Bring her face, her laugh into your mind. Take some slow deep breaths. As you inhale, gather all the love and positivity you possibly can into your mind. As you exhale, send all that light her way, see it shine down on her like sparkling twinkle lights... surrounding her, supporting her, soothing her. And you.

13 Weeks, 3 Days

It seems that this phase in life is full of challenges. And they just keep popping up, one right after another. The beginning of a pregnancy is full of tests and drawing blood and risk analysis. You can't help but get a little caught up in what ifs. And right when you've cleared one potential risk, another test, abnormal result, iron deficiency, who knows, seems to spring out of nowhere!

In order to at least *try* to not go completely crazy with worry, I'm trying to practice taking life *one day at a time*. You have no control over tomorrow; you have no control over the tests that have already been taken. Pregnancy is a constant practice of living in the moment *more* and learning to worry *less*. It's as if God is already priming us for the chaotic honor of being a parent.

So as you go about discovering the adventures of today, *Be Present*. Control the things you can, and learn to let go of the ones you can't.

13 Weeks, 4 Days

Take a moment. In the first seconds of the day, take a moment. Whether you're standing in your kitchen, sitting on a patio, or still snuggled into a cozy bed, just take a moment. Close your eyes and reach for the delicious hope that every new day brings.

I am blessed. I am strong. I am grateful. Repeat these words in rhythm with a steady breath and feel peace soak in. Your body feels light as the soul lifts to carry you through this day.

I am blessed. I am strong. I am grateful.

It only takes a moment…

13 Weeks, 5 Days

In the next few months emotion starts to rule our world. You might not necessarily be hormonal, but all thought and feeling, good and bad, are just below the surface of our maternal glow. You are learning to navigate a new life, a new chapter. Is it causing some chaos? At work, in love, with friends...no one really understands what you're feeling except you. And maybe your other mama friends. It was essential for me to find a way to calm my mind and master my emotions. The only alternative to that was to become more introverted. That can work for a little while, but eventually the need for community wins out. So what else can help? Meditation? Church? Yoga? Therapy? A much needed girls' night out with some movie popcorn? Living in the moment is the only true solution.

"You can't stop the waves, but you can learn to surf."
~Jon Kabat-Zinn

Learn to surf. Learn to ride the waves of yourself.

13 Weeks, 6 Days

Guess what tomorrow is, little mama? It's a cause for celebration, that's what it is! Tomorrow is the start of your SECOND TRIMESTER! A majority of women report feeling much better during the second trimester, and that's a reason to rejoice, right? The fog of fatigue lightens, and we begin to feel more like our old selves. Energy returns and nausea eases. And mentally, we enter a new phase. One step closer to meeting our baby. Make sure to toast yourself tonight with some sparkling apple juice. Send the first trimester on its merry way, and dive head first into this exciting new time. Everyone will know soon enough the secret you've been keeping!

Second Trimester

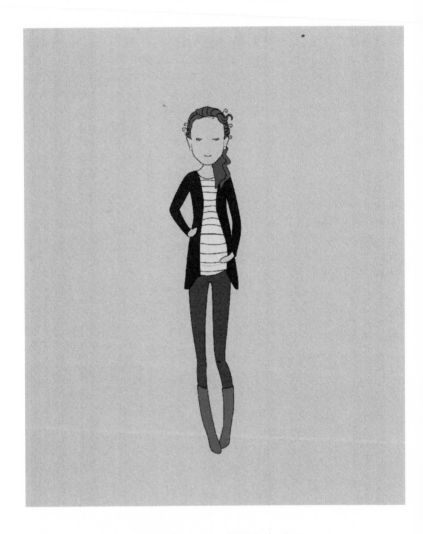

Week 14 – Week 27

The Daily Soul Sessions For The Pregnant Mama

14 Weeks

Sometimes life can overwhelm a person. It seems to overwhelm even easier when your hormones are raging and you're fighting for sanity every day during a time of enormous change. Outside elements, people, emotions can threaten this little calm world that you are trying to create. Tears are always annoyingly close - it's so hard to control your once controllable reactions. I find myself frustratingly close to snapping, saying something I regret, or letting my emotions take over more often than I ever did before.

But the truth is that our lives are simply a product of how we *think*, how we *perceive* events that happen around us. The only thing that we can control is how we *react* to the good, the bad, and the fantastic in this life. If I find myself spinning out of control at something that *happened* to me, I have to try to stay in the present. I have to remove myself, close my eyes, and take a few deep breaths. I don't want to be an over-emotional woman. A woman who is way too sensitive to other oblivious people in the world. I want to be strong. I want to be graceful. I want to be inspirational.

And so I am.

14 Weeks, 1 Day

Meditation: Finding Control

You must let go of the past. You must let go of regret, sadness, jealousy, and the what ifs. You have to learn to ruthlessly tear them out and scatter them to the winds. They have no place in this life you are working toward. No place in the life of the sweet little babe inside of you. Memories, sure, take memories with you, but all the chains that connect you to those memories that might hold you back must be broken...and vanished forever.

Close your eyes and bring one negative emotion or memory to mind. Something that is bothering you, nagging at your skull that you want to take control of. A secret, perhaps...one that only you know. Feel it like a ball of energy in the palm of your hand. Now take a deep breath and simply blow the ball away. Like the seeds of a dandelion, scatter that emotion to the winds. Take control. *You have control* of every thought, every emotion that takes root inside of you. It's powerful. It's beautiful. It's confidence. It's today.

14 Weeks, 2 Days

Pregnancy Around The World: In Latvia, godparents take a very active role in the child's life. In fact, parents believe their children inherit their *godparents'* good qualities. The godparents even choose the unborn child's name...so make sure you choose wisely!

14 Weeks, 3 Days

"Almost everything will work again if you unplug it for a few minutes, including you."
~Anne Lamott

Ain't that the truth. One of the best things I learned from my mother was to pick your battles wisely. Not everything is worth fighting over. She taught me to take a breath, unplug from my emotions so I could gain perspective and truly decide if this fight is worth it. Most of the time it isn't. Time heals, time soothes, time fixes everything.

14 Weeks, 4 Days

We all just need more magic and spirit in our lives. It's that simple, really. What inspires you? Causes you to dream? Keeps you faithful? Puts a smile on your face that starts deep down in your soul? Is it the ocean? An artist? A favorite book? Sometimes I get bogged down in the daily routine, and I have to stop and remember what fuels my inner pilot light. If I get distracted from that, I feel it in a negative way. But honestly we should never feel "stuck" during this incredibly "unstuck" time in our lives. Never before have we experienced this much daily change...

Ignite that pilot light today...what are you waiting for?

14 Weeks, 5 Days

Let me let you in on a secret, Mama. Life is precious. *All* life is precious. Why is it that we are so good to our growing babies, our partners, everyone else in our lives, but not to ourselves? Comparison, judgment can take seed in your mind and you become so *unloving* to yourself. Work on being nicer to you today. Work on forgiving yourself today. Work on praising your incredible body for all the work it is doing today.

...All life is precious. That includes yours too.

14 Weeks, 6 Days

"Don't believe everything you think. Thoughts are just that - thoughts."
~Allan Lokos, <u>Pocket Peace: Effective Practices for Enlightened Living</u>

If people could read every thought I had throughout the day, life would be a messy, messy affair. Thank goodness all our insecurities, moments of weakness, and silly fears can be kept to ourselves...most of the time. Don't give too much weight to your negative thoughts - they are so heavy it is hard to ignore them. Follow the light...literally...follow your light thoughts today as they lift you into a world of possibility. And then fly.

15 Weeks

***Mindfulness**: a mental state achieved by focusing one's awareness on the present moment, while calmly acknowledging and accepting one's feelings, thoughts, and bodily sensations, used as a therapeutic technique. (Oxforddictinoaries.com)*

Every day is a chance to work toward this one thing. Being mindful. Nine months of pregnancy seems like a long time. But like everything in life, this too shall pass. So the goal is to "calmly acknowledge" every bird, every gust of wind, every bad thought, every ache in the joint, and just accept today for what it is. The 105th day of this pregnancy, and one more day you are alive.

Make it a good one.

15 Weeks, 1 Day

Ever heard of the phrase *fake it 'til you make it*? Or how about pasting a smile on your face when all you want to do is frown. They say a person who even forces a smile on blue days will *ultimately be happier* than the person who sulks the hours away. Because the smile *will win out* in the end. That's a fact.

Meditation: Mantra

On days when you feel the emotions and hormones of pregnancy to be difficult, try this technique: Choose a word - any word that inspires you - and make it your mantra for the day. What could it be? Strength, grace, passion, love...close your eyes, take some deep breaths and repeat your chosen word as many times as you need. Breathe until you feel the strength, the grace, the calm seep in and carry you through this blessed day.

15 Weeks, 3 Days

Boy…girl…boy…girl…

Whether you're having one baby, or twins, (or - gulp - even more), this mystery is a constant and consuming companion of yours. Some of us find out early, some wait longer, either way it is a nail biter that won't go away!

Enjoy that feeling of expectation. Smile in wonder at the butterfly anticipation! What other surprise is as exciting and full of possibility as this one?

Boy…girl…boy…girl…

Seek out other pregnant women. It's a lovely and entertaining club you are now initiated into…if you let it be. Shrug off unwanted advice or chatter that doesn't suit you, and focus instead on the friends who inspire you, the friends who make you laugh your way through this often hysterical adventure.

There is nothing better than a good belly massaging and soul smiling laugh. And if it makes *you* feel this good…imaging how the little nugget is feeling too.

15 Weeks, 5 Days

What are you afraid of today? Fear can motivate us, paralyze us, piss us off, or just exhaust us. What are you afraid of today? Stretch marks? The health of the sweet baby growing inside you? Perhaps it's a fear of losing the life you led before. It could be a million different things, but for today, for right now, pick one. Pick one fear and dwell on it for just a few moments. Acknowledge this fear to yourself, your heart and soul, and watch what happens.

Life will always be full of challenges sowing seeds of doubt that creep in to hinder you on your journey. The more we can see these fears - identify with them, let them have their moment - the easier we can begin to breathe through them…and send them on their way.

What are you afraid of today?

15 Weeks, 6 Days

Change. That's what true fear is. Some form of change. But change is inevitable in this life, and if we can't get a handle on it the fear will win. And that is unacceptable. So. Change. Bring it on. What small thing could I change today just to prove I can? My hairstyle? The usual way I drive to work? How about a workout? If I try something new, and change just a little, maybe I'll master this fear of the unknown.

Even if it's just for today.

16 Weeks

Balance: *a condition in which different elements are equal or in the correct proportions. (Google Definitions)*

What part of your life (or body!) is out of balance at this moment? Take a step - even a small one - and correct it.

Journal Exercise: pull out your journal and spend some time writing. Start each sentence with *Today I will...* Finish as many sentences like this as come to you. Taking some control back and deciding *I will* can be a very powerful balancing act.

16 Weeks, 1 Day

"All that I am, or hope to be, I owe to my mother."
~Abraham Lincoln

As you continue on this journey to motherhood, send a little love and light to your own mother. She walked this very path - in these very footsteps - with you. It's illuminating to think about the circle of life and how truly enduring it is. Mom. It's a role so many have. And now you get to have it too.

16 Weeks, 2 Days

Being grateful immediately releases your mind from negative focus. Some days are harder than others to stay light. The hormones can so easily take over and take control, and to what purpose? When I feel a negative thought begin to win out, I immediately start to mentally list all the things I am grateful for. From the love of my husband to the smallest lavender plant in my garden…I change my thoughts. And my focus shifts. Every time. Whatever was bothering me cannot survive in these happy conditions.

16 Weeks, 3 Days

Fighting fatigue is a daily struggle in some - all?! - stages of pregnancy. The second trimester is filled with more energy and less sickness, but you're still tired. So tired. Has it been a stressful, busy time? Holidays, work, family vacations... maybe just a few consecutive days that have kept you on your feet constantly.

I find my body gets so tired after these times, and all I want to do is lie down and sleep for a few days. The motivation to begin moving again is hard. But we have to, mama-to-be. My yoga mat is calling my name - what's calling yours? I choose an energy boosting prenatal class that is filled with breath and movement to send the fatigue out of my body. Because the energy is there…it's just waiting underneath layers of sluggishness.

So get up and do something you love to get that energy moving. Meditate, walk, salute the sun with a grateful smile. You are literally *filled with life* right now. It's a heady thought.

16 Weeks, 4 Days

Meditation: Finding Energy

The sun puts out enough energy every second of every day to keep this planet alive. Surely you can use some of that energy today.

Step outside and find that sunshine. Lift your face to its warmth, and feel the beams of energy that shine down on your shoulders, your cheeks, your eyelids. Imagine those waves of sunlight filling all the space inside you. Let that sunshine energize you from the tips of your toes to the strands of your hair. Breathe in and out slowly, and be grateful for the sun, be grateful for the life that it gives to all of us today. Then see yourself as the sun to your baby. And be grateful for the energy that you are giving that life inside.

They say that in the days, months, and years after pregnancy we will look back on this time in our life as we look back on our childhood. Full of wonder, awe, and a wish that you had grasped and enjoyed every single fantastic moment of it. These nine months seem slow while we are in them, but in the story of our whole life…it is but a blink of an eye.

I challenge myself, and you, to take in the moments, the aches, the awe…and enjoy them all. Every single one. Create the memories that will stay with you for the rest of your life.

16 Weeks, 6 Days

Everything happens for a reason. Are you a person who believes in that? It's difficult on hard days to step back and truly accept that most things are out of our control. Most things just happen - and then it is up to you and me to decide how we choose to react. Every single day is a series of actions and reactions...and reactions during pregnancy seem to be supersized. So. Everything happens for a reason. Whatever happens today - let's strive to accept it with grace, faith, and hope.

Happy: *Enjoying, showing, or marked by pleasure, satisfaction, or joy. (Thefreedictionary.com)*

Every single person I know wants to be happy. As humans, we struggle and yearn toward that one state of being more than almost any other. That's the goal in life…to be happy.

"If you are jealous, you are living in the past. If you are worried, you are living in the future. If you are at peace, you are living in the present."
~Lao Tzu

And there it is. The secret to finding happiness. Living in the present. At all times, every minute, every day.

"The present moment is all that exists…most people live in a mental world. When we drop out of this mental world into the Now, we experience a depth, a richness, and a joy that feels sacred."
~Gina Lake, 60 Meditations for Greater Happiness

What greater time is there than now, when you're in a constant state of change, to practice living fully *in the moment.* Living fully *happy.*

17 Weeks, 1 Day

It is your 120th day of being pregnant! Yogis believe that the soul enters the body and becomes fully conscious on the 120th day…what a beautiful thought. Whether you believe in that or not, take a moment to cherish, bless, love your baby that is growing inside you. Sing a song, say a prayer, salute the sun, bake some cookies, do something with your full intention on your precious little one.

On the 120th day the soul enters the body…

…Can you feel it?

17 Weeks, 2 Days

In a way you are being more creative now than you ever have been before. You are the artist of a brand new life. Even though you aren't physically holding a paintbrush, a microphone, a camera, or a pen, you are building and nourishing and giving life to a brand new soul. How cool is that? Less than half the people on this planet can say that. So smile and give the world a little bit of that creative, beautiful knowledge today.

17 Weeks, 3 Days

Water. The elixir of life. Farmers pray for it. Native Americans have dances honoring it. 80% of a newborn's weight is made up of it. Sometimes we view rain as a bad thing - it gets in the way of whatever we have planned for the day. In reality, we should feel nourished by it, replenished, and washed clean. As mothers in the making, nourishment is very important when growing a baby. For the rest of our lives we will be providing the nourishment for our children. Milk, food, love, safety. Every time you drink that water today, instead of trying to "get through" those ounces, think about the nourishment you are providing. For yourself. For your baby. Water. The elixir of life.

Meditation: Nourishing Rain

Close your eyes and steady your breath. Picture yourself lying down outside somewhere - a forest, a field, a sandy beach - in the middle of a summer rain. A soft, cleansing rain that falls upon you like a thousand kisses on your skin. Focus on the nourishment that rain brings to the earth with every drop that spills from the sky. The rain heals you, rejuvenates you, gives you life. Absorb the life energy that this nourishment provides, and pass it along to the sweet baby sleeping inside. Breathe. And feel the rain...

17 Weeks, 5 Days

An American girlfriend of mine is living in England for a few years. She and her husband just found out they are pregnant - yay! - and it has been fascinating hearing her stories abroad. The one I found most interesting was what her OBGYN said to her on her first visit. She asked her what her expectations were for this pregnancy. More specifically, did she want a "European Pregnancy" or an "American Pregnancy." Suffice it to say I believe my friend went with "somewhere in the middle", but I was intrigued. How different our world takes on fertility, what you can eat, what you stay away from. It sounds like Europe is a little more lax on some points, and I'm fascinated. Prosciutto, cappuccino, yes please. Maybe I'll have bebe number two in the south of France…

Which would you choose? European or American? Either way, she'll be having her little prince or princess soon - which is really all that matters in the end!

17 Weeks, 6 Days

Life. What an interesting maze it is sometimes. We are filled with opposing feelings right now - the knowledge that you are invincible, strong, and your womb is safe. But at the same time you feel incredibly vulnerable, and that precious life inside needs you so. Be grateful today for your body. For your baby. For life. At almost 18 weeks this pregnancy feels like the norm - but it's not. It is but a fleeting time in your life. So treat yourself with a little bit of reverence as you go about this beautiful day.

18 Weeks

"Radical self-care is quantum, and radiates out into the atmosphere, like a little fresh air. It is a huge gift to the world. When people respond by saying, 'Well, isn't she full of herself,' smile obliquely, like Mona Lisa, and make both of you a nice cup of tea."
~Anne Lamott

Catch flies with honey. Kill 'em with kindness. Take the high road. Pick one and stick with it today. Don't let the small stuff getcha down.

86,400. The number of seconds you are given in one day. *This day.* The number of moments to make the most of today. How many wonderful things can be done with 86,400 seconds?

18 Weeks, 2 Days

Apparently we will start to feel the baby move any day now. Is that a butterfly? A worm crawling in your tummy? Indigestion? Ha. That fluttering sensation is one of the most exciting and unbelievable feelings you'll ever feel...at least up to this point.

18 Weeks, 3 Days

I've met two kinds of pregnant women so far: the ones that enjoy this time with unending abundance, and the ones that don't. The ones that feel a little subdued for the whole nine months. Hormones are as crazy as we are, aren't they? Sigh...it seems kinda unfair that we can't even medicate them with a nice glass or three of Sauv Blanc. But I digress. Mama - if you just don't feel like yourself, try to remember it won't last forever. And the gift waiting at the end is the most surprising and exciting one of your life. Whether that's the baby or the Sauv Blanc is entirely up to you...

Kidding...

18 Weeks, 4 Days

Everyday leads us a little closer to tomorrow and a little farther from yesterday. Isn't it amazing to think about your life 18 weeks ago? Like any year, I am always amazed at how much life *changes* over 365 days. Sometimes in big ways - a new house, a new job, a new *baby*. Sometimes in small ones - haircuts, favorite foods (did you know your taste buds change every seven years? My seven-year-old nephew informed me of this, and now I'll have to Google it. And try flan again, obviously). It doesn't matter the size of the change. All that matters is that life, people, the daily news - none of it - stays the same. We are ever flowing, ever moving on toward the next adventure.

18 Weeks, 5 Days

In my life, I have seen many sunsets. We love to romanticize that big golden globe as it sinks slowly out of sight. We enjoy it with friends, share pictures on Instagram, try and catch that magic flash of green that signals the end of the day. But how many *sunrises* have you caught in your lifetime? I could probably count them on one hand. It's interesting seeing as they are equally as beautiful as their counterpart, yet most of us are tucked sleepily in bed when dawn's rose-colored fingers make their morning debut. I read a blessing that said, *"May every sunrise hold more promise, and every sunset hold more peace"* (Blessing Unknown). It intrigued me. The sunset does bring peace. Peace that the day is done, and we made it through. But the sunrise? The sunrise is the promise kept. The promise that a new day has come. A new chance, a new start, a new hope for what *this day* will bring. It's a lovely thought as we bring a new life into the world. Talk about something to be hopeful for...

The less sleep I seem to get in this pregnancy makes me want to see more sunrises. How about you?

18 Weeks, 6 Days

Meditation: Journal Challenge

In the coming week, I challenge you to a writing meditation. For the next seven days, get up 15 minutes earlier and get out your journal. Spend those first, hazy, caffeine yearning moments free-writing whatever comes to your head. It might be mindless words, it might be a to do list, it might be a story, a song remembered, a diary entry. It might be a prayer. For the new day that is waiting. Whatever it is...clear your head of the clutter, and make room for an inspiring week.

19 Weeks

Reinvent: *change (something) so much that it appears to be entirely new. (Oxforddictionaries.com)*

Having a baby is a blank page. A fresh start. What dreams may come with a brand new life? It's a heady thought, but who doesn't love a new start? Maybe that's why every single person you see is so delighted and obsessed with everything about you right now. Have you noticed this? People are so filled with hope at the thought of a new life. A new dream. A new start.

It seems the perfect time to reinvent yourself as well. As you greet the morning, take a moment to ponder what ways you want to reinvent yourself, your soul. What kind of woman do you want the world to know? What kinds of dreams have yet to be dreamt? Until the day we die, we are a work in progress...and with a little bit of awareness, a little bit of love, that work can be inspiring.

Who do you want to be today?

The Daily Soul Sessions For The Pregnant Mama

19 Weeks, 1 Day

Meditation: Listen to the World Around You

Let's take in the world today - bring the outside in for a moment, and get out of our small world. I hardly ever take time to listen to the world around me. I'm too busy filling it with noise, to-do lists, and work. Try this meditation with me today:

Close your eyes and settle the breath. Do not quiet the mind, but open up to the elements around you. What do you hear? A car passing? Wind through the trees, a far away bark from a dog…Perhaps children laughing or a screen door slamming. Just people watch with your ears for once. It's amazing what you hear. Life is all around you: every day this world is filled to the brim with motion, adventure, routine, and nature. Be grateful today that you are one small but very significant part of this world.

Well hello belly button, it's nice to meet you. Kind of like the houseguest who overstays their welcome, I feel like my "new" belly button is here to stay. It's the ultimate pregnancy look, cute little belly popping out, even cuter little belly button just...out there...for the world to see. IS that cute? I keep changing my mind. One day I am elated by the growing, and the next...it can be a little stressful. It's hard to watch your body change so much and be completely out of your control. But this growth is temporary. Just repeat that when you find yourself worrying. It is temporary. What is inside will come out, and then that belly button will pop right back into its rightful, tiny, cute LITTLE place.

19 Weeks, 3 Days

We are well into the marathon of pregnancy now, and it's completely natural to think about what kind of mother you hope to be. Will you be the enforcer in your parent partnership? Enforcer or not, we all want to be the kind of mother that inspires and raises strong, self-aware children. But remember how we said yes to whatever our parents said no to? Where is the balance between strict and understanding? Sometimes I find it is more effective to bend a little than to be too rigid. It's a fine line that we will soon be walking...

"To be a powerful woman, you don't have to be aggressive or forceful. Like a tree, you have to find your roots and then you can bend in the wind."
~Angela Farmer, Yoga Teacher

19 Weeks, 4 Days

Pregnancy Around the World: The African Elephant has the longest gestation period known of mammals. They carry their babies for 660 days. That's 22 months. Um...The next longest mammals are the giraffe and camel, which come in at a measly 400 days. Just remember that when you feel like you still have a long road ahead of you. It could always be longer... (Scienceiq.com)

19 Weeks, 5 Days

At five months pregnant, your baby can begin to hear sounds outside the womb. Imagine that! In the next week, your little one will begin to perceive your voice, your partner's voice...the world outside! Start warming up those vocal chords and pick some favorite lullabies and Disney tunes...

Your little peanut will probably remember them once they are born!

"Everything grows rounder and wider and weirder, and I sit here in the middle of it all and wonder who in the world you will turn out to be."
~Carrie Fisher

20 Weeks

Halfway! You are officially halfway! What a milestone to be thankful for. Just enjoy that thought as you go about this day. Halfway!

Meditation: A Grateful Heart

They say that inside the womb is actually a very loud place. Your baby hears a lot of white noise with the steady beating of your heart above all else. That is why they are soothed by vacuum cleaners, dryers, sound machines, and your heartbeat. Let's meditate today on that heartbeat, and inject it with gratitude as it beats for that little one inside.

Close your eyes and let your mind drift. Mentally list all the things you are grateful for right now. This minute. I am grateful for the sunshine on my cheeks. I am grateful for the ocean outside my window. I am grateful for the roof over my head. I am grateful for the pancakes I ate for breakfast. I am grateful for the strength of this body. I am grateful for my husband...

Focusing on how we are blessed leaves zero room for anything negative. Light always beats the dark.

20 Weeks, 2 Days

The roller coaster of pregnancy never ceases to surprise me. I still struggle with comparing myself to the world and everyone in it. Being surrounded by pregnant women is inevitable, it seems that like continues to attract like. I am constantly amazed at the various stages of pregnancy and how it affects every single woman differently. We are lucky to have people to talk to, to share hilarious or alarming stories with, to be in the trenches with during this crazy journey. And I have to continually remind myself that my trials may not be your trials…but without a doubt, we *all* have trials of our own.

So I throw comparisons out the window like yesterday's trash, and enjoy this day, this moment, and whomever I get the pleasure of seeing.

20 Weeks, 3 Days

Intuition. Instinct.

My yoga practice has focused a lot on these two words this week. Yoga spends a lot of time working on the breath moving in and out of the body, helping to cleanse and purify as we stretch and strengthen our muscles. With that focus on inner awareness, it is much easier to tap into our intuition, and then that elusive *mother's instinct* we hear so much about.

The endgame in all this is that we become a mother, right? And with that, we are suddenly seen as caretakers, and all knowing figures in our children's lives. It's so strange, but if you take a moment, you can *feel* yourself starting to hone your intuition. It's starting to become easier and easier to say what you think, and feel how you feel, without worrying so much about the outside world. This must be because we are becoming mothers...

...and we are growing up right before our eyes.

20 Weeks, 4 Days

Advice: guidance or recommendations concerning prudent future action, typically given by someone regarded as knowledgeable or authoritative. (Google Search Definitions)

Are you as familiar with this topic as I am by now? Amazingly enough, advice will come out of the woodwork more and more as the weeks go by. Don't get me wrong, I love seeking and receiving as much advice as I possibly can before this baby arrives. However, sometimes it can overwhelm you. Especially when the baby registering begins.

So today my challenge for myself and for you is to just take a breath. When the opinions swirling around you become a little too much just take a breath. We've all been or are about to be first time moms; we will all "figure it out as we go". Like everything in life, you choose what works for you, and you forget all the rest.

…And when in doubt, a cup of mama-to-be tea and a nice romance novel will take all your worries away.

20 Weeks, 5 Days

I woke up this morning in a very introspective mood. Thinking about the future, about my life, and how it is going to change in ways I really can't even imagine. Sometimes I am excited by this change - ready for the next phase of my life. And other times...I am terrified by it.

What we can't seem to figure out is how we are going to feel before we feel it. Will you love your maternity leave and want to stay home forever? Or will you be itching to get back to work?

I know we can't predict the outcome, so we have to go with the flow until we find out. Because worry is such a waste of time...

20 Weeks, 6 Days

Is that baby inside a swimming fool yet? So far, I've heard the first feelings of fetal movement described as butterflies, effervescent bubbles, indigestion, and a worm wriggling just beneath your skin.

I think the worm describes it best so far - what do you think? Can you feel the tiny movement on the outside yet? How *cool* is that?

And we, as childbearing women and future mothers, are the ones who get to experience it. Try explaining that one to your significant other.

21 Weeks

"The call to adventure is the point in a person's life when they are first given notice that everything is going to change, whether they know it or not."
~ Joseph Campbell, <u>The Hero's Journey</u>

There are all kinds of adventures. Grand and dangerous ones, romantic and passionate ones. But what about the small seemingly routine ones? Just because we get used to something does not mean we shouldn't try to be inspired by it day after day. *Through the eyes of a child*...that's how I want to live my life. And you yours.

21 Weeks, 1 Day

"The starting point is realizing that letting go is not a dramatic moment we build to some time in the future. It is happening now in the present moment – it is not singular but ongoing."
~Judy Lief

Today is as good a day as any. Let go…and live.

21 Weeks, 2 Days

"Don't just pretend to love others. Really love them. Hate what is wrong. Hold tightly to what is good. Love each other with genuine affection, and take delight in honoring each other."
~Romans 12:9-10

Just a little inspiration as you go about your day today. We are all connected, from the smallest child to the oldest among us. I can be so closed off sometimes, in even the simplest daily chores - like going to the grocery store or dropping clothes at the cleaners. I want to be more open, more loving. Even in my relationships, I challenge myself to treat them as if they've just begun - with delight, spontaneity, and adventure!

21 Weeks, 3 Days

In this life, choosing to be happy is not enough. We have to see life through the eyes of a child, perceiving everything for the first time. Keep spontaneity and joy in your heart, so negativity and boredom cannot creep in. We have to change our perspective on life with all its joys and all its challenges. Find the adventure in everything and everyone, and you'll find peace and happiness in every moment.

21 Weeks, 4 Days

There is a tribe in West Africa where people do not count a birthday from the day of birth, or conception even. When a woman of this tribe decides she is ready to have a baby, she goes off into the wilderness by herself and sits down in nature. There, she composes a song. About her hopes, dreams, and wishes for the child she is ready to bring into the world. That is the day the baby is "born". Once the song is complete, the woman will go back to her village and teach it to her partner. They sing this song from that point on, conception, pregnancy, birth…this song becomes the theme for this child, sung at all major events for the rest of his or her life. The song is one of a kind - unique - lovingly made for that one soul. (Thoughtcatalog.com)

Beautiful isn't it?

21 Weeks, 5 Days

Pregnancy is a time to step away from the analytical side of our brains and embrace the primal one. The miracle of changes that we get to experience right now is ancient. The secrets and mysteries of carrying life have been passed down from woman to woman for millions of years, and it's special. It's awesome. It's bigger than we can really comprehend.

It the most creative thing we ever get to be a part of. Congratulations Mama...

21 Weeks, 6 Days

Meditation: Through the Eyes of a Child

Do you remember being a kid? Everything was so easy, so simple. Life consisted of the next game, the next adventure. I loved my bedroom. It had big windows with a huge oak tree outside that changed color with the seasons. In the summer it housed birds singing. In the winter it was silent and mysterious with snowfall. Either way...it was peaceful.

Close your eyes. Remember a memory from your childhood. Something you loved, somewhere you felt safe, some game that inspired you. Let your soul fill up with that innocent and hopeful feeling. Sometimes it is so restorative, so magical to see life through the eyes of a child. Try it today.

22 Weeks

This morning I came across this statement by Dr. Stephan Cowan, a 25-year veteran pediatrician:

"The secret of life is letting go."

I was instantly intrigued, instantly drawn in by this statement. I've been focusing a lot on *change*, and how we can accept the constant *inconsistency* in our lives with more grace and beauty. And I loved looking at life this way. He goes on to say:

"Life is a process of constantly giving way. Things pushed past their prime transform into something else. Just as spring gives way to summer, so is each stage of development a process of letting go. Crawling gives way to walking. Babbling gives way to speaking. Childhood gives way to adolescence. By breathing in, you breathe out. By eating, you poop."
~Dr. Stephan Cowan, *Fire Child Water Child*

HA. So true and I just loved this! Dr. Cowan is obviously focusing more on life after our child is born, but it's great food for thought today.

…The secret to life is letting go…

What do you need to let go of today?

22 Weeks, 1 Day

I have decided that comparing ourselves to other pregnant mamas may be one of the worst symptoms we experience in these nine months. And now is the time it can get really ugly. As our amazing tummies start to pop, every single one of us is different. It is so hard to simply let go and just enjoy. Enjoy the amazing organ that is our uterus and never, not once - *ever* - compare ourselves to someone else. And yet we do. So many of us waste precious seconds, minutes, hours on feeling not good enough, not skinny enough (we are *pregnant*, eh hem), that our bodies aren't changing the way we want them to…

"There is no other organ quite like the uterus. If men had such an organ they would brag about it. So should we."
~Ina May Gaskin

You and me…we are experiencing a miracle. Enjoy being a part of the miracle.

22 Weeks, 2 Days

Why is it so much easier to focus on the negative than the positive? I bet if you kept track, way more good things happen to you in one day than bad. And yet that one negative comment or encounter can haunt you for days. If you find yourself in this boat, try to focus your energy elsewhere. In an interview with CNN, the Dalai Lama was asked what the first thing was that he thinks of in the morning. He replied, *"shaping motivation"*. He said everyone must *"be vigilant so intentions are focused in the right direction"*. Focus outward, not inward. Focus on kindness, not hate. On compassion instead of jealousy. Shape your motivation today, Mama. You only have today - so how do you choose to live it? (Ed and Deb Shapiro, Oprah.com)

22 Weeks, 3 Days

This morning, before the day's crazy takes hold, give yourself one moment to focus outward. If you journal, write down three names of people in your life that could use some extra love today. Then add two or three simple things you could do that might help those souls out. A handwritten letter maybe? A phone call, flowers left on a doorstep...an invitation to coffee - the possibilities are endless. Focus outward today. You and your sweet babe will feel the difference!

22 Weeks, 4 Days

Baby moon. Who knew this was a thing? Don't get me wrong, any kind of moon - honey, full, baby, or blue - are full of surprises. And I like surprises! What kind of trip would you enjoy right now? The whole point is to spend time with your love before - what? - you never see each other again because you're both way too busy with your 2.5 kids, dogs, school, sports and goodness knows what? It all sounds a touch dramatic, and I have strong to quite strong hopes that my husband and I will rise above this cliché. But I'll take the baby moon regardless. Bring it on!

Now. Where to go?

22 Weeks, 5 Days

It continues to amaze me how different every pregnancy is - yet at the heart of it - how very, very same. I know we all handle the ups and downs differently. Some women retreat and hibernate, others seek out as much companionship and as many hobbies as possible. The one thing I have learned throughout this season in my life is the laughter and pleasure of your friends will trump hibernation any day. So if you're like me, don't give in to the isolation all the time. Make an effort to go to that prenatal yoga class, meet a girlfriend for a glass of - um - lemonade, go see a hilarious chick flick. You weren't meant to feel alone in this. So don't.

22 Weeks, 6 Days

Meditation: Let Go

Close your eyes and settle your breath. Place your left hand on your heart, your right on your belly. As you inhale, think of something you want to let go of. A regret, an argument, a worry, a mistake. As you exhale, imagine that regret leaving your body just as the breath does. Visualize all your negative emotions and thoughts literally exiting your world as a feather is carried away on the wind. Sometimes my mind will get stuck on one thought, and I spend the entire meditation repeating that one worry, until finally, finally it releases. Releases me. And frees me.

23 Weeks

"Everyday is a winding road...I get a little bit closer to feeling fine."
~Sheryl Crow, Singer-songwriter

This song was stuck in my head when I woke up at the crack of dawn today. I haven't heard it in years and yet there is was. So simple. So hopeful. So deliciously cliché that it must be true.

"Everybody gets high, everybody gets low. These are the days when anything goes..."

23 Weeks, 1 Day

"This is the day the Lord has made. Let us rejoice, and be glad in it."
~Psalm 118:24

This day is perfect. For some, it is a day of challenges - others a day of success. Whatever came before, whatever comes after...

Be glad in today.

23 Weeks, 2 Days

Has the baby shower mania begun yet? Registering for this new life is...challenging shall we say? How are you supposed to know how many breast pads to register for? There are so many strollers, swings, diapers, and bottles out there. Asking you to choose them now is like asking you to make a chocolate soufflé without the recipe! (mmmm soufflé...). If this were a game show, I'd immediately use a lifeline and phone a friend - someone who's been there, done that, and knows which products worked best for her. God Bless all the Mamas out there...

It really does take a village.

23 Weeks, 3 Days

I swear I've never seen so many pregnant women and strollers in my life until I joined the pregnancy club. Isn't that crazy? We don't notice what is not a part of our lives. It makes me wonder what else I am missing everyday. Perhaps today I will consciously *open my eyes* and see the world around me. I bet there are countless beautiful moments to be a part of...right now.

23 Weeks, 4 Days

Isn't it amazing how much this pregnant belly changes throughout the day? I feel so light and airy in the morning and so heavy and stretched out by the time the sun goes down.

It's morning right now. I better go enjoy this lightness - cuz that baby will make itself known any minute.

23 Weeks, 5 Days

Meditation: Happy Place

Phew my emotions are just *bubbling* under the surface these days. Are they for you? It's a little frustrating to deal with sometimes. You just start crying for no reason. The tiniest thing can set you off in a tailspin of sadness. Thankfully we get to blame these annoying and slightly uncontrollable outbursts on hormones. Or at least I do.

BUT. I still dislike them. I still want to create a peaceful environment for myself, for my hubby, for this sweet little baby. So how do we do that? It seems Jim Carrey had it right - *find your happy place*. Take a moment amidst all the chaos and emotion, and find some solitude within yourself. Close your eyes. Take deep breaths. Imagine yourself in the one place that always brings a smile and soothes, and stay there in your mind for a minute or two. When you open your eyes, carry that peace with you, and be the calm, strong, fierce woman you want to be.

...Virgin margarita anyone?

23 Weeks, 6 Days

Stillness: *Silence, quiet, hush. (Dictionary.com)*

What a challenge it is these days to find stillness in our lives. It seems an oxymoron: How do I achieve stillness on the outside when my insides are in a phenomenal state of *busy*. It is so easy to ignore my yearnings for stillness and just get swept up in the daily drama, challenge, blur and bustle.

Yet I crave it. I don't function as well without it. My heart silently whispers to me to slow down for a moment, find the stillness, so I can appreciate this beautiful day.

Find that stillness, even if it's just a moment of it. Let it steady and strengthen you right now. Right now.

24 Weeks

Your sweet little baby is now technically able to survive outside the womb. With lots of medical help, of course, but congratulations! What a milestone to cherish and celebrate today! Perhaps a sip of champagne, a massage, or a dance in the kitchen with your love is just what you need. You deserve it!

24 Weeks, 1 Day

Intuition: *the ability to understand something immediately, without the need for conscious reasoning. (Google Search Definitions)*

Think about this word today. To understand something *immediately*. No delay. Intuition is a part of you, simply *of you*. Just like this baby growing inside you is *of you*. They say we develop a mother's intuition as this process progresses. I look forward to it.

24 Weeks, 2 Days

Listen*: to pay attention to someone or something in order to hear what is being said, sung, played, etc. (Merriam-Webster.com)*

As I start this day, I want to start it with an intention. I want to work on my ability to listen. To my husband, to my friends, and most importantly, to myself. To my body. To this life that is growing inside of me. It is a vital skill that I so want to extend to my child as she grows up. From newborn to young adult, I want to listen. It's a loving act, full of respect for the people around you. To give someone your time and attention…to listen…

…Imagine all the wonderful things you'll hear.

24 Weeks, 3 Days

Visualize this day without judgment.

What would you do? What would you say? What kind of dreams would you decide to go for today? It's amazing the different kinds of judgment that hold me back from realizing my deepest dreams - big or small. Not just judgment from others, but judgment from myself.

So. Today I choose to live without it. Endless possibilities await. Fantastic adventure. Passionate living…you choose it…

…and live it.

24 Weeks, 4 Days

As you awaken to this brand new day, Mama, let us awaken to the authentic side of ourselves. The natural, primal, *female* side of us is where our intuition lies. It can be easy to drown that out and forget how to hear the completely natural and organic signs within our body.

In your morning musings, yoga, or workout, take care to truly listen, and hear how your body is responding to the day. Respect yourself, and let the emotions and adventures of this day wash over you like cool, cleansing water.

Meditation: Positive Affirmation

As you lie quietly in bed and prepare to get up and greet the morning, set an intention for yourself. Can you hear your lover's quiet breath beside you? Or feel a delightful kick from your baby inside? Before we begin this day, let these precious moments fill us with gratitude, with grace.

Today I am inspiring, creative, and joyful in everything I do.
Today I am inspiring, creative, and joyful in everything I do.
Today I am inspiring, creative, and joyful in everything I do.

What is your intention today?

24 Weeks, 6 Days

I've found myself more introverted this week - really this month - than usual. Have you noticed changes in yourself? I try to accept this and let the need for quiet and calm just be what it is. Part of me still wants to hold on to the old me, the habits that I used to have. It can be hard to simply accept who I am right now. Today I find I am soothed by a good book and a cup of hot chocolate.

What soothes you today?

Worry is inevitable. For some reason, it always hits me in the mornings. That seems to be my quiet time, when my soul wanders, and worries tend to creep in. Worry is a part of life I'm learning, and I'm also finding that if I cannot learn to cut these infectious thoughts out of my head, they will take root, grow and only do damage to my sanctuary. To my home and my family. Feeling grateful and taking a moment to remember my incredible blessings is the best warrior I have against worry. I use it with joy and gratitude, and every time I win. Worry cannot stand against Grace. It cannot survive. And I can live this day in peace and love.

25 Weeks, 1 Day

Meditation: An Exercise in Gratitude
Write down action words that are a part of your life. Right now. Free flow your thoughts and see what wonderful things already exist in you today. Here was mine this morning…

I love. I live. I inspire. I motivate. I laugh. I rejoice. I dance. I sing. I write. I create. I eat. I pray. I do. I cherish. I give. I learn. I see. I seek. I read. I wonder. I travel. I discover. I cook. I participate. I help. I listen. I feel. I relax. I enjoy. I run.

…I begin.

25 Weeks, 2 Days

Do you have time to read, busy Mama-to-be? I just finished *Bringing Up Bebe* by Pamela Druckerman. Now that you are 25 weeks, the reality of actually bringing a child into this world and raising him may be settling upon you with more weight every day. This book follows one mama's journey of raising her children in Paris. It was a funny and very interesting read on the differences in parenting styles across the ocean. You may find it stimulating, intriguing, and, oooh la la, so French.

25 Weeks, 3 Days

Pregnancy around the World: In Belgium, the health of mama and baby are numero uno. Their goal is to keep the mother stress and ache free, so they prescribe massage - that the insurance companies cover!

Hmmmm I'm a fan of Belgium now, and the moral of the story is *go get a massage*! It's good for you, it's good for the baby, and it feels amazing.

25 Weeks, 4 Days

It's hard to believe that in 101 days there will be a new little boy or little girl in this world. A little one that you and your love *created*. I get used to the daily routine of pregnancy, the discomfort, the attention, the kicking, all the strange symptoms. But the one thing I have not gotten used to yet? It's the one thing that all these symptoms and routine are leading toward...

A new life. A new baby. A new beginning.

Sometimes I just have to remind myself of this...and maybe it'll sink in tomorrow...

25 Weeks, 5 Days

Has the insomnia hit yet? I have been "blessed" with sleepless nights this week. What a lovely way nature has of preparing us for the sleepless nights to come.

As usual, life is all about how we perceive it. The one good thing I take away from the long hours in the night is the fact that this baby inside has been holding one man dance parties to keep me company. It never fails to bring a smile to my face. What good can you wring out of the bad today? It'll help to ease the trouble and stress of the week.

25 Weeks, 6 Days

Has motivation been a little sluggish? Getting on that treadmill, visiting your yoga mat, even putting on makeup or tight maternity jeans seems like a chore as we get bigger and bigger...and bigger. So where can we find the motivation? How can we tap into the wells of energy within us that seem to be hiding these days?

The old saying *one foot in front of the other* comes to mind today. Even if it's just a prenatal stretch or restorative yoga class online, your baby and your body will thank you for it.

26 Weeks

"In the end, only three things matter: how much you loved, how gently you lived, and how gracefully you let go of things not meant for you."
~Buddha

Just a sweet thought to carry with you today...

26 Weeks, 1 Day

Allow: to permit (someone) to go or come in, out, etc. (Merriam-Webster.com)

Literally. This is what we are doing every single day. It's a blessing, and we have made this choice to *allow* our bodies to become a sacred vessel. Rejoice in the fact that you have the ability to *allow* your body to accept this baby and nurture him for the rest of his life.

26 Weeks, 2 Days

Allow: *to give the necessary time or opportunity for. (Google Search Definitions)*

As your body quite literally takes control of you, you have to work every day to *allow* that dictatorship to happen as gracefully as possible. Let go of trying to accept your disappearing waistline, and just *allow* it to happen. For now.

It will be your turn again…someday.

In order to accept what your body is going through, your life must become a daily workshop in letting go. Isn't that the basis for change? Letting go of something or someone in your life and moving forward to new somethings, and new someones.

What thoughts do you need to let go of today? Figure it out, and Let. Them. Go.

26 Weeks, 4 Days

In Native American culture they call the full moon Grandmother Moon. She is healing and wise, full of advice and a careful word. Be conscious of the lunar cycle and let the next full moon soothe you, bring you knowledge and peace to the awesomely ancient changes that are happening inside of you.

Meditation: Moon Meditation

The moon. Like other mysterious, orbiting objects hurtling through space it can make you feel small, insignificant, humble… Or it can make you feel peaceful, and give you relief that you are you, and anything that happens in this world is not as big as that moon…

Close your eyes. See that silver moon in your mind. It willingly changes shape before us every month, shrinks to almost nothing at all, and then expands to its brilliance once again. Without resisting. Kind of like you right now, Mama. Breathe in and out, expand and shrink, take in and let go. Don't resist this growth in your life. If the moon can do it…so can you.

26 Weeks, 6 Days

What is in a name? Do you know what your name means? Strong, Brave, Graceful, Adventurous... Do you feel it's your identity? Has that changed the way you've approached your life? Or has it not affected you at all? Have you thought of baby names yet? What a privilege, what a responsibility it is to name someone. Whether you find out the sex of this little nugget or not, it is fun to talk about names. After all, it will be theirs forever. Just as yours is yours. So. What does your name mean?

27 Weeks

Have you attended a baby class yet? They aren't for everyone, but my husband and I went to a newborn class this week. We both decided that it surprisingly made us feel secure in the knowledge that we actually knew more than we thought we did.

So much of this whole process is instinctual. If we can just keep tapping into that inner knowledge, then motherhood becomes the logical next step in the storybook of our lives. And we can approach the coming months with confidence and calm…or try to at least.

27 Weeks, 1 Day

It's inevitable for the mind to turn toward thoughts on labor and delivery at some point in the last few months. I've been struggling for inspiration in this battle of body and will that is my reality right now. I found this:

"And once the storm is over you won't remember how you made it through, how you managed to survive. You won't even be sure, in fact, whether the storm is really over. But one thing is certain. When you come out of the storm you won't be the same person you walked in."
~Haruki Murakami

Are you feeling a storm coming on? Try to accept it. The warrior within all of us is always ready to take over…and she will, when the time is right.

27 Weeks, 2 Days

Do you remember how carefree you were as a child? How confident and fearless and filled with dreams just bursting to come out! It never occurred to us *not to* dream - one, two, ten, *twelve* dreams a day were perfectly normal.

"Sometimes I've believed as many as 6 impossible things before breakfast."
~The Queen, Alice in Wonderland

Future Mama - we are about to raise our own dreamers. Such a hopeful thought. I want to be a mom who leads, not just by teaching, but by *doing* as well. So. Today I choose to dream. All day long....and make one of those dreams a reality. Even if it's just a small one! Play dress up, be a famous chef for the day, sing at the top of my lungs and convince everyone I'm a Broadway Star!

What's your dream today?

27 Weeks, 3 Days

Meditation: Find a Class

Do you have 10 minutes this morning? Here is my encouragement for this day. Find a quiet spot in your home and meditate for 10 minutes. Today I visited Yogaglo.com and chose a 10 minute meditation on happiness. It was a lovely way to start the day. Being present. Being happy. Being alive.

27 Weeks, 4 Days

Light a candle for your little one this morning. While you enjoy your single cup of coffee or a cool glass of water, set your mind on the flame and let it represent the precious little baby inside you today. Send a good thought and set a good intention for you and your passenger...and let that take you through your adventures today.

27 Weeks, 5 Days

As I stare the third trimester square in the face, I find myself a touch dismayed today. I don't like to focus on negative feelings, but sometimes I have to acknowledge them before I can send them on their way. As the tummy gets bigger…and bigger…and bigger, it can stress me out rather than give me joy. I know I am creating a miracle and a growing tummy is required…but sometimes this is hard to remember. My old, *younger self* creeps in (an oxymoron if you think about it), and I feel a small sadness at the demise of my seven month-ago body. My seven month-ago life…

Phew. I said it. Are you feeling this at all? Don't be afraid to acknowledge the sad sometimes. This is a truly awe inspiring, emotional event in our lives - it can't *always* be good. And as I write this, I feel better for having put it out there. Now I can deal with the sad, and get right back to the glad…like the Reese's Peanut Butter Cup I'm about to eat.

27 Weeks, 6 Days

"Be not the slave of your own past - Plunge into the sublime seas, dive deep, and swim far, so you shall come back with self respect, with new power, with an advanced experience that shall explain and overlook the old."
~Ralph Waldo Emerson

This was the perfect quote to come across after my musings of yesterday. Be brave. Be bold. Life, as you know it, has forever changed.

Third Trimester

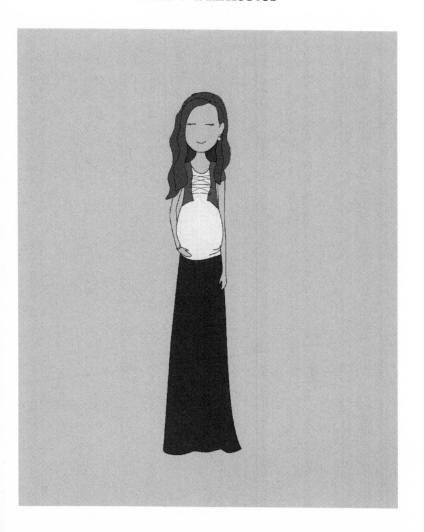

Week 28 – Week 40...and beyond!

28 Weeks

THIRD TRIMESTER!! Oh my gosh how did this happen! Congratulations Mama!

"Remember how far you have come, not just how far you have to go. You are not where you want to be, but neither are you where you used to be."
~Anonymous

…Ain't that the truth?

28 Weeks, 1 Day

Nesting: To create and settle into a warm and secure refuge. *(Thefreedictionary.com)*

We've heard this term before. Expecting mamas nest. That's what we are supposed to do during the months we wait for this baby to arrive. I always found myself shying away from that term. It sounded so homely, kind of boring, and a little controlling. What did it mean anyway?

Now I find myself much more introverted than I ever used to be. The growing symptoms of pregnancy demand it in some ways. We get tired quicker, and our body doesn't want to do the things it used to. There is so much going on inside, you can't help but draw in on yourself during these last few months.

I'm coming to terms with this. Like a blazing fire that pulls at you on a chilly winter night...I've decided *nesting* is just what it says it is. Making your home into a *warm and secure refuge*. For you, for your husband, for your child - a place that is alluring and safe. And peaceful for all.

Meditation: Moonlight

Close your eyes. Visualize a bright full moon shining down on a peaceful lake at night. Visualize yourself floating down this sparkling moonlit path - the light infusing you with peace and wisdom. A wisdom that is much more ancient than you or the new life you're creating. Find stillness and let the moonlight teach you patience today.

28 Weeks, 3 Days

Pregnancy Around the World: In Korean Tradition, the mother must give the news of her pregnancy in a certain order; first to her mother-in-law, then her husband, and finally her own mother. Soooo…who did you call first?

28 Weeks, 4 Days

"The only man I know who behaves sensibly is my tailor; he takes my measurements anew each time he sees me. The rest go on with their old measurements and expect me to fit them."
~George Bernard Shaw

Ha. This takes on new meaning in the second half of pregnancy. Change is inevitable. Even if it's your dress size. Not to worry...it can change again.

28 Weeks, 5 Days

Morning Exercise: Do something creative today. Take time to write in your journal, paint a new picture for the baby's room, dance in your kitchen, try a recipe you've never made before - whatever your creative spirit desires - *give into it*. So much of your energy is pulled toward that life inside. It's nice to take a few moments of the day and focus on the life outside.

"If I had my life to live over, instead of wishing away nine months of pregnancy, I'd have cherished every moment and realized that the wonderment growing inside me was the only chance in life to assist God in a miracle."
~Erma Bombeck, Author

29 Weeks

Dream:

a: *a series of thoughts, visions, or feelings that happen during sleep*
b: *an idea or vision that is created in your imagination and that is not real*
c: *something that you have wanted very much to do, be, or have for a long time*
(Merriam-Webster.com)

Frightening. Seductive. So beautiful it makes your very soul ache to think about. You become nostalgic over something that hasn't even happened yet. The fear of missing out. Wanting to run but having no idea where to go. Time is passing too fast, and if you don't move you will never ever get it. That is what it is to dream.

29 Weeks, 1 Day

"To everything there is a season…"
~Ecclesiastes 3

And every season has its challenges, its joys, its fears, and its tempo. Let the rhythm of this season take over. Don't try to control your days, but slip into your emotion like you slip into a lake on a hot summer day. Sometimes squealing…sometimes breathless…always relieved.

29 Weeks, 2 Days

Well…it's happening. Perhaps the hormones are getting stronger and stronger, or perhaps we are just mourning the loss (or gain?) of another 10 pounds on the scale. Either way, the tears and emotions are so close these days aren't they? Try to ride the wave of feelings as best you can, but don't hold it in. If you feel like crying, cry! Let those salty tears cleanse you from the inside out - you will feel washed clean, and you will breathe so much easier after they pass.

You are so strong! A warrior Goddess does not have to ignore her feminine, emotional side. It is learning to cope and to ride these waves that make us stronger and fiercer in the end.

29 Weeks, 3 Days

Good morning Mama-to-be! As we greet the day, look for joy in the little things. Let's try to live *reactively* today. Instead of treating this day as a blank page, with nothing planned or predestined, how about you *respond* to this day. Take in and notice all the blessings that *happen* around you. Everyday the Divine Spirit, God, and Creator fills this world with millions of tiny gifts for you. A sunrise does not bring a blank page. When we open our eyes to actively receive these gifts, our whole perspective - *our whole world* - can change.

29 Weeks, 4 Days

I am a believer in positive affirmations. Whether it's to state out loud the things I am grateful for, or a quick pick me up before a nervous situation, they make me feel powerful, happy, and strong. However...

"When we ask the universe for something, the unspoken message is that what we want does not exist, and the universe accepts this as truth."
~Madisyn Taylor, Author and Founder of Daily Om

Instead, our affirmations should state, not ask, our desires as if they *already exist*. It's a strange way of thinking about the things you want in life that you do not yet have. Yet Taylor goes on to say:

"When we affirm that we are fulfilled rather than deficient, we are asserting that contentment is a natural way of being."

Then like attracts like, and the universe will follow.

How do we state positive affirmations as if they already exist? It's more than just putting an assertive spin to your thoughts - it is truly believing in your dreams, in yourself, before they are actual reality.

"Ask yourself how you would feel if your wishes were granted, and then allow yourself to internalize that emotional state."
~Madisyn Taylor, Daily Om

The idea is that if we can find that emotional state, truly feel it in our bones, then the universe recognizes it as reality, and your visions as fact! So. What affirmations about this baby, your new life, can you believe today? It's a whole new world.

Meditation: Positive Affirmation
I am strong, I am beautiful, I am life. I am strong, I am beautiful, I am life. I am strong, I am beautiful, I am life...Keep going Mama. Keep going.

29 Weeks, 6 Days

I thoroughly encourage you to talk out loud to your baby these days, Mama. Even more than yourself talking, encourage your husband or partner to as well. There really isn't a sweeter moment than in the early morning hours or late at night when your man rolls over and speaks sweetly to the little one inside.

Love, gratitude, and an overflowing sense of cuteness for your partner will come over you. It's seriously the most adorable thing to see.

30 Weeks

Another week down! Only 10 more to go…food for thought today:

Have you considered looking into a prenatal corset/girdle for after you give birth? Many prenatal yoga teachers, doulas, and childbirth coaches recommend them to help stimulate your stomach's muscle memory and return it to your pre pregnancy shape. My Prenatal yoga teacher, Patricia Grube (Serenitybirth.com), suggests you start wearing it 24 hours after birth.

Girdle…here we come.

30 Weeks, 1 Day

"If you wait for perfect conditions, you will never get anything done."
~Ecclesiastes 11:4

Ok Mama...what are you putting off in your life right now? Perhaps you have finally started maternity leave, or this trimester has simply forced you to slow down a little, put your feet up more, and rest your busy body. This is *the perfect time* to do a little dreaming, a little goal setting, a little scheming for the future. You are already starting a brand new chapter in the adventures of your life...so...what else do you want to throw in there to add a little character. Add a little spice. Go on - you're the writer - *create it.* And then do it.

30 Weeks, 2 Days

"Comparison is the thief of joy."
~Theodore Roosevelt

Ponder that as you start this day. It's been an ongoing theme for me throughout these past seven months - comparison. Such a wasted emotion. Teddy had it right.

I choose joy.

Meditation: Finding Joy

Think of something joyful. Or just think of the word *joy*. Can you feel it in your belly? That effervescent energy rising up through your heart, your head, the tips of your fingers until it's bursting out of your pores. It's fleeting and fantastic. But that is it. That is joy. And I bet you're smiling right now.

30 Weeks, 3 Days

The days get longer as sleep starts to elude you now. They say it's nature's way of preparing for sleepless nights once the baby comes. Or it's simply the fact that we get up to pee 14 times a night. Either way, you may have more time on your hands.

Take up a new hobby, if you can. I found painting incredibly soothing the last few weeks. It doesn't matter if you aren't an artist. Simply have fun with paint, tap into your inner child, and put color on canvas. The hours melt away and you'll find some peaceful moments to keep you company.

30 Weeks, 4 Days

Look into purchasing a delivery gown for your time at the hospital. The standard hospital gowns are so scratchy and uncomfortable. Check out www.PrettyPushers.com for some in-style labor wear! They have all the right openings for monitors, IVs, and epidural access.

30 Weeks, 5 Days

"It is not only that we want to bring about an easy labor, without risking injury to the mother or the child; we must go further. We must understand that childbirth is fundamentally a spiritual, as well as a physical, achievement. The birth of a child is the ultimate perfection of human love."
~Dr. Grantly Dick-Read, 1953

It seems important to remember that childbirth is not just a scientific, medical event we are about to go through. It is spiritual, ancient, and innate. It is *Love*.

A woman holds stress and anxiety in her hip joints. So it is natural to assume that how you are feeling toward labor and childbirth is reflected in how sore your hips are. The tension will pool, collect, and become stagnant...trapping all those negative thoughts inside you.

Combat these feelings and free up anxiety by stretching out this area. Try pigeon pose, or cobblers pose to help you release tension today. Breathe in peace and courage, focusing on the hip joints. Imagine this cleansing breath swirling and soothing around the tension. Then acknowledge the fears and worries that are out of your control and breathe them out...sending them far away, sweeping the achiness with them. And leaving peace and calm in its wake.

31 Weeks

"All of my life, in every season, You are still God...and I have a reason to sing....I have a reason to worship."
~"The Desert Song" Hillsong

31 Weeks, 1 Day

Mamas. I heard a new term today. *Labor down.* It involves the stations your body goes through towards the end of labor and using that information to help your doctor determine when's the best time to start pushing. It is so important to educate ourselves. Talk with your doc about your hopes and expectations now while you have the time. I still have so much to learn - don't we all?

31 Weeks, 2 Days

Meditation: Balancing the Worry

What steps can you take to balance out the worry of labor and childbirth? Worry is such a wasted emotion…what sense does it make to get all worked up over something that hasn't happened yet?

Try this next time the butterflies and stress start to spiral out of control…

Close your eyes. Witness the worry. Breathe deeply and stay in the present moment. Place that worry inside a bubble, and as you exhale, send the worry bubble on its way. With every exhale, send the bubble further away. Watch as it gets smaller and smaller, until all you're left with is a cool, clear, calm breath.

31 Weeks, 3 Days

Restless, restless soul. Are you feeling the pull of it? Perhaps slight boredom, an urgency to get to the next phase of this pregnancy but powerless to make time go faster. One answer is yoga. Find a prenatal class in your area. Connecting and being around other pregnant mamas is soothing in it's own way. Or take a class online. Whichever - breathing and meditation can help to contradict that treading water feeling right now.

31 Weeks, 4 Days

Trust in the process. Look around you...sometimes you can feel so isolated during these nine months. From your friends, in your body, from your old life. It can feel like you are all alone and perhaps the only woman to go through pregnancy. But you are not alone. Countless women have walked in your footsteps, felt the growing pains and the panic at what's to come. Take solace in that fact. If they can do it, you can do it...you just get to put your own sassy mark on it.

She thought she could...and so she did.

31 Weeks, 5 Days

In Kundalini Yoga, it is believed that your baby isn't born with her own aura intact. Mama shares her aura with her baby: that is why they say to keep your little one close for the first 40 days. In fact, your aura has the capability of expanding to nine feet around you, and some cultures believe that the mother should never be further than that from her newborn for those 40 days!

31 Weeks, 6 Days

In Astrological terms it is the Age of Aquarius (and will be for about 2100 years) - and an age for fierce mamas. You are your baby's first Guru, or teacher. So be strong today and know you will teach your little one epic love and lifelong courage. They say it's the best job in the world.

32 Weeks

"When you have come to the edge of all light that you know and are about to drop off into the darkness of the unknown, FAITH is knowing one of two things will happen: There will be something solid to stand on or you will be taught to fly."
~Patrick Overton

Two months to go!

32 Weeks, 1 Day

Is that little bundle of joy kickboxing inside you yet? It is so remarkably awesome to observe how much you have changed in the past eight months. If it doesn't pain you too much, take a moment to look at some pictures of yourself from right before you found out you were pregnant. And then give thanks for this miracle that is growing inside of you.

Then use that picture to motivate you for getting that booty back…in a couple more months!

32 Weeks, 2 Days

"You must understand the whole of life, not just one little part of it. That is why you must read, that is why you must look at the skies, that is why you must sing and dance, and write poems and suffer and understand, for all that is life."
~Jiddu Krishnamurti

And that is why you must find the awe in your journey *right now*. You are a sacred vessel these nine months. Such a short time really. Glean and scrape, experience and memorize every single terrifying and lovely bit of it.

32 Weeks, 3 Days

Meditation: A New Day

With every sunrise comes a chance to be exactly who you want to be. Yesterday may have had its stresses, it may have brought its aches and pains, but that's the magical thing about today. It's a new day, and you get to do with it whatever you wish.

Take a mindful breath. Visualize the sun rising. See the horizon. See the golden ball of light getting bigger and brighter with each moment. Feel the warmth on your face as the sun takes its rightful place in the sky. Smile. It's a new day.

32 Weeks, 4 Days

"Fear of the future is such a silly disease."
~Jedidiah Jenkins, Author

Embrace, love, look forward to, be fear-LESS of the future...

32 Weeks, 5 Days

We cannot bring to the world what we don't have within us. Or think about it this way: we cannot teach our children what we haven't yet learned. If you want to raise a peaceful child, you have to learn how to cultivate peace within yourself. If you want to raise a confident child, you have to learn to master confidence within yourself.

It's so simple, yet it feels like constant chaos, doesn't it? We are a never ending work in progress - don't stop learning and changing, so you can bring the best to the next generation.

32 Weeks, 6 Days

These last few weeks bring so much internal focus. Sometimes this causes me to forget about the outside world and selfishness takes over. One amazing way I've learned to combat the depression or anxiety that follows is through *service*. Serving others, volunteering, helping out a friend in need - by intentionally pushing the focus off ourselves and onto others - it is truly amazing how the anxiety can simply melt away.

Who can you serve today?

33 Weeks

"Who of you by worrying can add a single hour to his life? Since you cannot do this very little thing, why do you worry about the rest?
~Luke 12:25-26

Meditation: Learning to Deal with the Unknown

The next few weeks will be a study in excitement, apprehension, and suspense, and I find the butterflies are harder to control if I let my mind wander too far into the unknown. A quick meditation to slow my breathing, bring my heart out of my throat, and keep my mind calm has become necessary.

Wherever you are, close your eyes. Bring your left hand to your heart, and hold your right hand palm up, pointer finger and thumb touching. Start to breathe in and out, slowly deepening with each inhale. Take the tiniest pause at the top of each inhale, then one more at the end of every exhale. Continue for as long as you like. Feel how your body responds, calms, expands to handle every worry, every need. Repeat as often as needed. (Adapted from Kia Miller, Yogaglo.com).

33 Weeks, 2 Days

Distracting yourself may keep you sane during this last stage of pregnancy. Bonus points if you find a healthy way to do so! I'm looking at you, pancakes. Here's a fun one: Think of all the cheesy pregnancy movies that you watched before you were pregnant. At the time, we didn't truly understand what those women were going through. Guess what? Now you'll know every inside joke. So queue up Father of The Bride Part II or What To Expect When You're Expecting and have a movie marathon this weekend. You'll laugh and cry - ah that music in Father of The Bride - and it's not *so close* to your due date that the delivery will make you decide to keep that baby inside you forever. Remember, it's Hollywood! They take major dramatic liberties...right? *RIGHT?*

33 Weeks, 3 Days

Change. New beginnings. Journey. Any big life event comes with a strong dose of the unknown. Do you fear the unknown? Yearn for it? Revel in it? We just bought a house, and boy, is it an adventure. You go from complete exhilaration to suspecting buyer's remorse in less time than it takes you to walk up your new stairs. And then before you know it you are ecstatic again. Will you be happy there? Are your neighbors crazy? Was that paint color really the right choice?

It's hard to see the future - impossible actually - to know how you'll react to the sleepless nights, the endless feedings, the *being responsible for a new life*. No wonder we are kept up at night. No wonder our hearts are silently telling us to search out peace...to find ways to stay in the moment, stay mindful, stay happy...stay strong.

33 Weeks, 4 Days

If you could have one do-over this pregnancy - what would it be? I think I would have tried to enjoy my second trimester more. That was the bubble wasn't it? Finally less tired, finally less sick, and so smack dab in the middle of this whole thing you don't really think about the end yet. Well…now you do. How can you not? This train will arrive heart stoppingly soon, and you will have to get off it, Mama, no matter what you're feeling. There is an unexpected freedom in that though - the certainty that you have no choice. Like Christmas morning, the new season of The Bachelor, or a sunrise…it will come.

33 Weeks, 5 Days

I swear I've never been so ready to get out of bed then when I am pregnant. Are you suddenly and inexplicably a morning person? I used to love sleeping, love snuggling, love bedtime. Now it's like we are so exhausted from sleeping - I use that term *very loosely* - that we'll do anything to get the day started! Pregnancy insomnia is no joke, Mama, and it is frustrating. I've had to become a morning person just to fight back. Repeat after me: the early hours are peaceful. Dawn is the time for journaling, for sitting outside with a steaming cup of tea, for reveling in your *aloneness* before the hectic day begins.

33 Weeks, 6 Days

Curious*: Eager to know or learn something. (Oxforddictionaries.com)*

Are you curious today? To finally meet your little one? To find out what labor will be like? To discover who this unborn babe will become? To see if you can really lose that baby weight? To EVER have a normal, non-awkward sex life again?! It's enough to keep the days interesting, that's for sure.

> *"I think, at a child's birth, if a mother could ask a fairy godmother to endow it with the most useful gift, that gift would be curiosity."*
> ~Eleanor Roosevelt

Controversy. Life is filled with one obstacle after the next. It is how you view these obstacles and attack them that make you the person you are. I want to be a person who does everything with love, not hate or judgment. Starting with your birth plan and moving right on to parenting philosophies: no matter how different those are, we are all the same at the core. Parent. Mother. Woman. Sister. Be confident in your choices today, and then live this day with love.

34 Weeks, 1 Day

Why do some people accept change gracefully and others stick their heads in the sand and refuse to move on? Accepting big life changes is a delicate balance of finding solace in routine and being willing to let go. If you can do this at the same time, finding comfort in change (aka having a baby!) can be possible.

34 Weeks, 2 Days

How do we find a balance between letting go of the present and finding discipline at the same time? Discipline throughout the day is important. So that we don't become so overwhelmed by our changing circumstances, that we become scared and stagnant and get nothing productive done in the process. Yoga can offer the routine you are searching for. A daily practice will bring the spiritual and physical outlet for you to bring your worries and aches. The mat is a place to let all of that go. And live each day with grace and intention.

34 Weeks, 3 Days

Temporary: *lasting for only a limited period of time; not permanent. (Memidex.com)*

If there is one theme to focus on these last few uncomfortable weeks - it's that this is temporary. This will not last, and the next phase will come. The ebb and flow is constant, so we just need to breathe through this day...and get to the next.

34 Weeks, 4 Days

Meditation: This Too Shall Pass

Temporary. This too shall pass. Tomorrow is another day. To everything there is a season. Nothing lasts forever. Whether you are reveling in these nine months, or you're too excited to meet your little one to really enjoy them, take a moment to contemplate today. The discomfort, the hormones - they will go back to normal. The sciatic pain, the allergies, the sweating, the *whatever* - it will all go away soon. Even the feeling of being so close yet so far away from 40 weeks will pass. 40 weeks will come. And so will your baby.

Close your eyes this morning. Become aware of the breath as it travels in your nose, through your body, and out again. Over and over. Take in the new, let go of the old. The very air you breathe is temporary. This day, your cravings – they're all as fleeting as the breath inside your body. Keep breathing and feel the hope in knowing change is around the corner.

34 Weeks, 5 Days

Sleep. Such an elusive, fickle thing these days. But every once in awhile we receive a gift and sleep all the way through the night. If you lucked out, savor that moment of waking up in the first few moments of dawn. Give thanks, cuddle your love, and enjoy today.

It's the little things.

34 Weeks, 6 Days

In the moments before the rosy fingers of dawn light the world, your corner of the earth is in a state of waking. Just like you. There is a balance to the nature around you, and the hectic energy of people and daily life has yet to upset that balance. It's a lovely moment to spend meditating, praying, contemplating the incredible life inside of you. Feel the quiet, the peace, the calm...feel the hope and endless possibility that a new dawn, *a new life*, brings.

35 Weeks

35 weeks. 35 days to go. It's like our golden birthday of pregnancy. It may still feel like you have a few weeks to go, but when you put it in the perspective of days - it certainly seems exhilaratingly close.

35 Weeks, 1 Day

Do you wonder what your birth story will be? Everyone has a different one, and they truly never forget it. *This story* is a tale that will be told and retold your whole life. The excitement, the thrill, the breathless uncertainty - *this story* has all of that - in the best possible way. The best writers in the world can't make this one up. That gets to be your job.

35 Weeks, 2 Days

Meditation: Morning Mantra

Morning Mantra: Close your eyes, start to deepen your breath. Repeat: I am Strong. I am Fearless. I am Love. I am Strong. I am Fearless. I am Love. I am Strong. I am Fearless. I am Love.

"Birth is not only about making babies. Birth is about making mothers--strong, competent, capable mothers who trust themselves and know their inner strength."
~Barbara Katz Rothman

35 Weeks, 4 Days

It takes courage to do something you've never done before. A swallowing of butterflies, a banishing of insecurities - and a determination to try something new. *When was the last time you did something for the first time?* I heard that question the other day. Maybe if I try something new everyday it'll make me that much stronger for this HUGE "something new" that's coming. This takes doing something you've never done before to a whole new level.

35 Weeks, 5 Days

"You yourself are the eternal energy which appears as this Universe. You didn't come into this world; you came out of it...like a wave from the ocean."
~Alan Watts, Philosopher

Such as your baby comes out of you...and into their brand new world. Funny how they say we are all energy - it will take a tsunami of energy to get through the next month of your life. But you can do it. Energy is energy...and it is all around.

35 Weeks, 6 Days

Becoming a parent will probably include a lot of filtering our thoughts and watching what we say around the babes…and husbands…and mothers-in-law…and who else?! The world is not quite ready for complete transparency - but is this a good thing or a bad thing? I wish we could all just get along - isn't that the saying? Unfortunately, this isn't always the case. But as this day gets going, I'm going to send light and love to all my fellow mamas out in the great big world. No matter our beliefs, our styles, we are all the same at the core. We are all mothers…or will be very soon…

Meditation: Fear and Love

Fear and love cannot coexist. You must choose one over the other. So choose love. The middle finger is Saturn finger. The finger of challenges. Try this meditation: link the two middle fingers together, and pull apart with your elbows in line with your chest for the length of a song. This will strengthen you and help you with the process of letting go. Face fear, face challenges…and choose love.

36 Weeks, 1 Day

One reason why we already LOVE and are grateful to our labor and delivery nurses: They willingly work day in and day out, with emotional, hormonal, delightfully crazy mamas and papas to be!

So take a moment, even though you don't know her yet, and send gratitude to your nurse. You'll meet her soon enough.

Breathing is natural…it is one thing no one but God can take away from us. So always breathe, in the midst of chaos, remember to breathe.

36 Weeks, 3 Days

I woke up thinking what a chaotic, crazy, and cool event this is in the scope of our lives. The event of having a baby. All nine months of it. I want us to be up to the challenge. I want our whole worlds to shift, have new meaning, make us better people...amazing mothers! I still want to dream, you and I, but today I want us to be *renewed* in this *brand new life*!

Is that too much to ask?

36 Weeks, 4 Days

Time right now has a very fluid, very fickle meaning. You have less than four weeks to go, yet you could go at any moment (ah!). So it feels breathlessly close one minute, and years away the next. It's hard to get a grasp on the uncertainty of that, and I bet you've never packed for anything this early in your life!

36 Weeks, 5 Days

They say expect the best, but prepare for anything in childbirth. Educate yourself on all aspects of labor: natural, drugs, C section, whatever! That way you are prepared for any curve balls that are thrown your way, and you can handle them with grace and calm.

36 Weeks, 6 Days

Wait: *To remain or rest in expectation. To stay in one place or delay action until a particular time, or until something else happens. (Thefreedictionary.com)*

We are supposed to teach our children the art of waiting. The ability to handle frustration with maturity and patience. Right now we need to practice that art as well. This...waiting...this circumstance that is totally out of our control. The last month overflows with waiting. How can you find contentment in that?

37 Weeks

"How you approach birth is intimately connected with how you approach life"
~William Sears, <u>The Pregnancy Book: A Month-By- Month Guide</u>

Ah, and what does *that* reveal to you, Mama? There is still time to make new choices today. Approach today with a positive, light, and love-driven attitude.

37 Weeks, 1 Day

Down to the last few weeks. As they say, there are the first eight months of pregnancy - and then there's the last. No one really tells you about it, or how to prepare for it. But it will get challenging. It will get exhausting. It will seem never ending. After eight months of change, how can our bodies possibly change even more? And can you approach it with courage and humor? Because that is much more fun than the alternative.

37 Weeks, 2 Days

Meditation: Changing Gracefully

*"Yoga allows you the compassion to observe your weaknesses. Surrender your ego.
Let your best self walk through this day."*
~Jo Tastula, Yoga Instructor, Yogaglo.com

What honest changes can you make in your attitude right now? Make today a constant meditation. Be gentle with yourself as you mindfully observe any weakness. We cannot grow into better human beings until we accept where we are weak and allow ourselves to change gracefully.

37 Weeks, 3 Days

"Two things prevent us from happiness: living in the past and observing others."
~Anonymous

Just look ahead mama…there ain't no going back now.

37 Weeks, 4 Days

Only change begets change. The world slows down right now and tedium can truly set in, leading you to believe that this phase in your life will never end. It will though - maybe God makes this last month so challenging, we will cease to be afraid of labor and actually start to look forward to it!

37 Weeks, 5 Days

Get honest with yourself today. What do you project to the outside world? Is it the same as what you actually feel on the inside? Wouldn't it be a relief to feel exactly as happy and free as you want to show the world? It's so hard right now, because you are probably feeling huge, uncomfortable, and anxious of the future. So show that side to the world too! And then you can let it go and make room for a little peace.

37 Weeks, 6 Days

Buoyant*: able or apt to stay afloat or rise to the top of a liquid or gas. Cheerful and optimistic. (Google Search Definitions)*

Remember what feeling *light* used to feel like? Oh, to be floating atop a vast and refreshing lake. Close your eyes and remember how that felt. In order to float, the body must completely let go. Avoid sinking to the bottom through struggle and control, and rise to the top of peace and serenity today. Trust the process, Mama.

38 Weeks

"Remember this, for it is as true as true gets: Your body is not a lemon. You are not a machine. The Creator is not a careless mechanic. Human female bodies have the same potential to give birth well as aardvarks, lions, rhinoceri, elephants, moose, and water buffalo. Even if it has not been your habit throughout your life so far, I recommend that you learn to think positively about your body."
~Ina May Gaskin, Ina May's Guide To Childbirth

38 Weeks, 1 Day

The Core Chakra. The first of the seven major Chakras located at the base of the spine. It represents security, belonging, and finding your place in the world. As you move toward this new life, you might be struggling to find *your* place in the world. In your tribe. In your body.

Meditation: Core Chakra

Close your eyes and focus a red light surrounding your tailbone. Stand in Mountain pose and imagine red clay supporting your feet as they firmly plant into the ground. Continue to visualize a healing, energizing red glow around your tailbone. Intentionally balancing the first chakra can help you face this *new* life with courage and balance today.

38 Weeks, 2 Days

One of the best things you could do in the coming weeks is to find a body of water. God forbid it's summertime out there because you already feel like a human furnace. But search out a pool, a lake, a large Jacuzzi tub and sink in. Just float for a while and bask in the forgotten feeling of lightness. Weekend plans? Absolutely.

38 Weeks, 3 Days

Have you packed your hospital bag yet? Don't forget music and speakers to soothe and get your mind right. Battery powered candles add a lovely glow to combat the harsh fluorescent lights, and pillows from home are a must. Order your Pretty Pushers Labor Gown - you won't regret it. Just think - this may be the craziest trip you'll ever pack for!

Patience is a virtue. Isn't that the saying? The endless effervescence inside you changes rapidly from anticipation to terror, and it's tempting to pull back and hole up somewhere until this is all over. If that's today, then let it happen. We all become temporary introverts at some point during pregnancy, especially when the countdown begins!

38 Weeks, 5 Days

Gratitude time: Take a few moments this morning to close your eyes and reflect on the last nine months. You are probably feeling so heavy - in more ways than one - and it is extremely therapeutic to try and *lighten up* your world.

Finish this sentence: "Today I am grateful for..." What beautiful blessings are you thankful for right now? Forget about yourself for a moment and lighten your load Mama...

38 Weeks, 6 Days

If you haven't found a prenatal yoga class yet, try to now! Even one or two classes with other women going through the same thing as you can be very enlightening. Yoga can also help maneuver your pelvis into the optimal position for labor. It's a mind, body, and soul massage that will change your day!

39 Weeks

80% of women deliver between 37 - 42 weeks. That may seem like a small window of time...UNTIL you're the woman living through those five unbelievably long weeks. At this point in pregnancy a day seems like a year. Sleep is a thing of the past, you're peeing every three minutes, joints ache, and you simply feel like a giant breeding vessel that is focused on one thing only: *Baby*. Some mamas handle these last few weeks with grace and poise, not really caring when they go into labor and more than happy to let nature and baby do as they will. Some women - like me, eh hem - not so much. The waiting and anxiety seem endless. But it will end. Just tell yourself that...over and over if need be. This too shall pass.

"It is only through labor and painful effort, by grim energy and resolute courage, that we move on to better things."
~Teddy Roosevelt

The finish line is so close. You can do this!

39 Weeks, 2 Days

Labor: *to strive, as toward a goal; work hard. To move slowly and with effort. (Thefreedictionary.com)*

These are among the many definitions of *labor*. It's been a nine month marathon, and you are on the last lap. Unfortunately, it'll get harder before it gets easier, but all good things are that way. The good news is you're probably so tired of this dreaded tenth month that you may actually start to look forward to the last step!

39 Weeks, 3 Days

"Nothing is impossible. The word itself says I'm possible!"
~Audrey Hepburn

Stay strong Mama. It will happen. It will start. It will be incredible. It will be worth it. It will. It will. It will…

"I'm not afraid. I was born to do this."
~Joan of Arc

39 Weeks, 4 Days

Are you feeling alone in this stage of your journey? Like you are the only one going through this right now? Food for thought:

Roughly five children are born every second around the world. (InCultureParent.com)

Over three million women are pregnant at any given time in the United States. (Based on facts from the <u>CIA World Factbook</u>)

So if you are feeling down right now, chin up. You are most definitely not alone.

Meditation: You Are Not Alone

Get comfortable, precious mama, and close your eyes. If there are any other women in your life who are pregnant, bring them to mind. If you don't know anyone specifically, rest assured that there are a lot of other women in the world right now going through the exact same thing you are. Even though you don't know their faces, call them to your mind anyway. Say hello. Feel the powerful force that is enveloping you right now. This is a sisterhood, this is motherhood. Strong, powerful, beautiful, patient, loving. This is your clubhouse.

39 Weeks, 6 Days

"You gain strength, courage and confidence by every experience in which you really stop to look fear in the face. You are able to say to yourself, 'I have lived through this horror. I can take the next thing that comes along.' You must do the thing you think you cannot do."
~Eleanor Roosevelt, <u>You Learn by Living: Eleven Keys for a More Fulfilling Life</u>

Not that labor is "horror" per se...but you see what I'm getting at...

"Relax your shoulders and relax your heart. Let go and make room for the pain to pass through you. It's just energy. Just see it as energy and let it go."
~Michael Singer

Remember that your breath is your best friend right now! Each inhale leads to an exhale, and so on and so on. Connect the breaths, and you'll be on the other side of pregnancy before you know it.

40 Weeks, 1 Day

Meditation: Laugh It Up

You're ready. I know you're ready. Your partner knows you're ready. Your doctor knows you're ready. However, your baby may *not quite* be ready to say hello yet. The only thing you can do is laugh. I'll repeat that, the *ONLY* thing you can do is laugh. So start laughing, right now. Out loud! Laugh and laugh and laugh until the people around you start giving you *the look*. They may think you're losing it. But it's ok, because honestly, you probably are losing it. Just a little bit. Keep laughing, Mama!

40 Weeks, 2 Days

Spicy food. Sex. Castor Oil. Walking. Nipple Stimulation (you heard me). Will any of them bring on labor? Are they just old wives' tales? Have you tried curb walking? Here's how you do it: Find an open stretch of street that has a curb. Walk along the road with one foot on the curb and the other foot on the street below. Up, down, up down. You may actually look as ridiculous as you feel. Trust me, I tried it. And yes, I looked and felt ridiculous. But guess what!? I also laughed. Waiting is close to impossible these days, and laughter takes the edge off.

40 Weeks, 3 Days

Patience: *an ability or willingness to suppress restlessness or annoyance when confronted with delay. (Dictionary.Reference.com)*

A *willingness* to suppress restlessness - look at that. Are you willing to ignore the restless side of you?

> *"Patience is bitter, but its fruit is sweet."*
> ~Jean-Jacques Rousseau

You are almost there.

Nothing lasts forever, including this, I promise you. Think about it - your childhood? Barely remember it. Eighth grade? A blip on the radar. College? Blink of an eye. Pregnancy will end. You will become a mother soon. So tell yourself that today as you go about your business...

Nothing lasts forever!

40 Weeks, 5 Days

Lateness is not a virtue. Is there any situation in this world where being late is a good thing? They are few and far between, but come to think of it, your period being late is what started this whole adventure - actually another act started it, but you know what I mean - and that was a good thing! So let's think about the word *late* as a means to an end right now. This baby knows what she's doing, and in her mind, she's not late. She's right on time.

40 Weeks, 6 Days

It's just another day, Mama. Just another glorious, beautiful, magical day! I know you may not be feeling your tip top shape at the moment, but truth is truth. It is just another day. So distract yourself today and go see a movie, or get your nails done. Call a friend - your funniest friend! - and have her make you laugh. Go for a walk and really absorb the nature around you. Tilt your face to the sun, and feel its rays soaking into your skin. Enjoy this glorious, beautiful, magical day.

41 Weeks

"In this way, every birth is a natural birth: each of us is part of nature, not separate from it, and nature is always stunning in its variety. Your birth, then, is part of the natural world, however it unfolds."
~Lauralyn Curtis

"Nature is always stunning in its variety." Strong words. True words. Your story is stunning. Your birth story will be stunning because it ends with your precious and beautiful baby.

41 Weeks, 1 Day

"I am thankful for my struggle because without it, I wouldn't have stumbled upon my strength."
~Alexandra Elle

If there is ever a time to dig down deep, find strength, courage, and patience, now is it. You can do this. That baby will come at the exact right time she's supposed to - apparently our children begin to teach us things even before they are in our arms.

41 Weeks, 2 Days

Invincible: *Too powerful to be defeated or overcome. (Google Search Definition)*

THIS is a time for warriors. For positivity. For grace. These times of frustration, distraction, and anxiety can only be kept at bay with strength and calm. Like a mountain standing still and secure in a storm - you can be strong too. You can ride this storm out to the beauty and joy that's waiting on the other side. You are invincible.

41 Weeks, 3 Days

Is induction your least favorite word yet? My mother in law went three weeks overdue with her first. *Three weeks.* Apparently her body is incapable of starting labor. You learn something new everyday.

41 Weeks, 4 Days

Every object in motion stays in motion. Newton's first law. Keep moving, Mama. Keep moving.

And they all lived happily ever after - that's my mantra today. My life is a fairytale. A very large, very hot, very hormonal fairytale.

41 Weeks, 6 Days

"Sometimes it takes balls to be a woman."
~Elizabeth Cook, Songwriter

Amen.

Our Deepest Thanks...

Writing a book of daily inspiration turned out to be a lot like writing a song. Trying to capture a little magic using a short amount of words, and looking for that magic everywhere, every day, in everyone. First and foremost, I have to thank God for the love, grace, and opportunity I have been blessed with in this life. Being a creative soul takes a lot of courage and an endless amount of faith, and no matter what happens in life - *You have to keep being creative* - in whatever way you can. I'm so grateful that my sisters, Kate and Kara, jumped on board with this book as soon as I found the courage to tell them about it!

Together we want to thank our families. Our husbands - Rossi, Jason, and Billy - you are amazing husbands and bad ass fathers, and we couldn't get through one day without your love and support. To our mom, Genie, and our dad, Frank - you have taught us what family means. Family is sitting down together every night for dinner, it's 40+ years of marriage, it's being fantastic Grandparents to this new generation of kiddos. We love you guys more than words can say, and we thank you for encouraging us and allowing us to go after every dream we can possibly come up with.

Last we want to thank all our fellow mamas out there. From every amazing pregnant woman we sweat next to in yoga class, to our best girlfriends in the world - you inspired every page of this book. Like I said - Pregnancy isn't new to the world, but it is new to *you* - and every day should be just that. *New*. A celebration. Life.

About The Authors

Kacey, Kate, and Kara are sisters and mamas who love to cook, drink Italian wine, make music, and unexpectedly have babies within months of each other. Kate and Kacey are Grammy nominated songwriters and recording artists. Kara is a passionate blogger and photographer with experience in PR and marketing for the fine arts. They love to follow their dreams whether it be writing books, singing on the radio, doing a headstand in yoga class, or finally living in the same city at the same time. They currently reside with their husbands, kids, and dogs in Redondo Beach, California and Denver, Colorado. You can follow their adventures on Instagram and Twitter @thedailysoulsessions, @kccoppola, @kcleiva, and @karaschmahl.

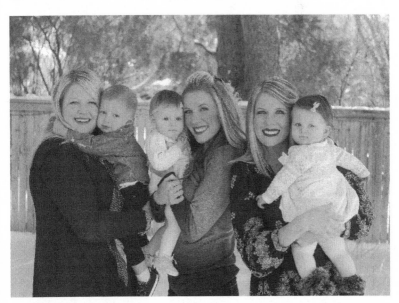

About The Daily Soul Sessions

Join our Tribe! We are passionate about making dreams come true.

We are committed to light and love and finding joy in Every. Single. Day.

www.TheDailySoulSessions.com

Instagram @thedailysoulsessions
Twitter @dailysoulsesh
Facebook @thedailysoulsessions

Made in the USA
Columbia, SC
06 July 2017